Aura

A Practical Guide to How to See Feel & Heal the Aura

(How to Charge Your Energy Field With Light and Spiritual Radiance)

Paul Decastro

Published By **Tyson Maxwell**

Paul Decastro

All Rights Reserved

Aura: A Practical Guide to How to See Feel & Heal the Aura (How to Charge Your Energy Field With Light and Spiritual Radiance)

ISBN 978-1-7772550-3-9

No part of this guidebook shall be reproduced in any form without permission in writing from the publisher except in the case of brief quotations embodied in critical articles or reviews.

Legal & Disclaimer

The information contained in this book is not designed to replace or take the place of any form of medicine or professional medical advice. The information in this book has been provided for educational & entertainment purposes only.

The information contained in this book has been compiled from sources deemed reliable, and it is accurate to the best of the Author's knowledge; however, the Author cannot guarantee its accuracy and validity and cannot be held liable for any errors or omissions. Changes are periodically made to this book. You must consult your doctor or get professional medical advice before using any of the suggested remedies, techniques, or information in this book.

Upon using the information contained in this book, you agree to hold harmless the Author from and against any damages, costs, and expenses, including any legal fees potentially resulting from the application of any of the information provided by this guide. This disclaimer applies to any damages or injury caused by the use and application, whether directly or indirectly, of any advice or information presented, whether for breach of contract, tort, negligence, personal injury, criminal intent, or under any other cause of action.

You agree to accept all risks of using the information presented inside this book. You need to consult a professional medical practitioner in order to ensure you are both able and healthy enough to participate in this program.

Table Of Contents

Chapter 1: Indigo 1

Chapter 2: Emotional Engagement 14

Chapter 3: Lavender With Physical Reality 31

Chapter 4: Finances And Profession Options 45

Chapter 5: Spiritual Values 63

Chapter 6: Finances And Career Options 76

Chapter 7: Highbrow Capabilities Of Humans Bearing White Aura 86

Chapter 8: The Science And Energy Of The Aura 105

Chapter 9: Reading Auras 131

Chapter 10: Harmonizing Your Aura 170

Chapter 1: Indigo

It is idea to be the youngest of all the Aura hues; it is said that the dynamics of the sector have been making fast adjustments, and it changed the dynamic power vicinity. With the alternate of environment, humanity is also growing and developing. These dynamics gave rise to new color - a coloration reflecting skills, competencies, and bodily characteristics great from all previous sunglasses. This new color includes all the capabilities and abilities required for human evolution.

The Indigo Aura is a message that encourages one to open their eyes and get out in their consolation location. It signs a time to take the initiative and chance and find out what opportunities are there for you. It symbolizes the want to diverge a incredible manner to face out and make others see what they need to offer. It's about being actual and comfortable in their personal self. The Indigo Aura speaks approximately love and kindness. It symbolizes compassion and peace. This colour seems in a single's air of mystery after they need serenity of their life. This color represents the need of their intelligence and notion certainly so proper motion can be taken.

It symbolizes the peace that one is just experiencing in their lifestyles or the need for extra peace in life. Moreover, you will be able to have a look at the traits of a fantastic leader or leaders with religious know-how.

Indigo air of mystery, people are loving, gentle, cute, and susceptible. There's a quiet electricity within the Indigos that allows them overcome personal worrying conditions, however it additionally carries a vulnerability in them that makes them enjoy matters at a deeper level. No one has to educate the idea of attention as they already have the knowledge about this. But the most hard a part of Indigos is to observe and growth endurance and tolerance. They want to recognize that the statistics they may be having remains to be superior with the aid of others, but occasionally they themselves struggle with this difficulty.

They are moderate, quiet, intuitive, and sweet in nature. They play a large element in reaching the stability and harmony that they certainly enjoy of their lifestyles. They don't run away from troubles at the same time as humans will count on them to do Instead, they to do subjects quietly and gracefully. They don't let all of us apprehend that they'll be prying a few components painful or tough. They don't need people to enjoy sympathy for them. They cope with their troubles within the terrific manner stated to them, and they don't want to comprise others in it. Just due to the fact they are very introverted, they may be satisfied to do their private matters by myself, and nobody asks them any question about that to provide help or refuses to go with them at the path.

They have this dependancy of wondering and stressful about lifestyles and seeking out methods to make it higher, making plans to triumph over the stressful conditions and frightening others honestly, and the way they want to satisfy their existence's motive. Indigo human beings are very curious ones, and they need to have complete records approximately how things paintings, They need whole statistics and information; that's why they recognize life in a better angle and feature answers to its mysteries At least maximum of them.

People also can keep in mind Indigos to be clever, however this is because of the truth they may be seeking to examine and assimilate new matters. They are just looking for to technique all of the data that is in their mind. They may probably look like calm and mild; however, they're expressive and unafraid to expose how they count on or experience. At a component whilst they are confident and apprehend they may be clearly right, they may be not going to move away it, and they may voice it out.

They are most willing to fight for justice. They can't see injustice taking place with anybody. They are a actual author that evokes sincerity, revel in, and hobby. They create what humans are although thinking, They are deeply inspired by means of the usage of their inner records, and this courses them to create the right choices and make the first-rate alternatives. They be given as actual with their instinct because of the fact they apprehend that it is their power, and it is are constantly proper.

Interaction of Indigo with Physical Reality

It has been observed that Indigo Aura human beings are extra touchy to energies, and that they react at enormously higher frequencies. Subsequently, their systems arrive at threshold all the more unexpectedly. This way that they get tired with out difficulty and early, and get stressed with too much noise. These intense energies or no longer on time incitement need to purpose them to pull lower again into themselves. Adults misunderstand this behavior as being rebellious, whilst the kid is trying to understand the emotional relaxation. This is due to a difference within the manner the biochemical systems of Indigos Aura shade were constructed. Parents want to apprehend this gadget for mutual blessings.

The high-quality detail about the Indigos is that they're born curious, and they want more, to find out. As they sense the change inside the frequencies round them, they may have sleep issues or awakened in nights with pains and ache.

The first connection with the Indigo Aura Color come to be accomplished in the year 1970 with the resource of a San Diego parapsychologist, Nancy Ann Tappehile her assessment determined a vibrational new colour that she had in no manner seen in advance.

In their ebook 'The Indigo Children', Mr. Carroll and Ms. Tober define the phenomenon. Indigos, they write, share developments like excessive I.Q., acute intuition, self-self warranty, resistance to authority, and disruptive dispositions, which might be often recognized as hobby-deficit sickness, referred to as A.D.D., or interest-deficit hyperactivity sickness, or A.D.H.D.

Indigo youngsters love dairy merchandise, however they're intolerant towards Cow's Milk, which causes better breathing troubles to them, like Congestion, Runny Noses, and ear infections. But they may be pinnacle to go together with Goat's milk.

The Indigo Aura machine is quite touchy to frequencies. So, they need a comfortable and serene environment. When exposed to extended instances of painful instigation, their sensory systems emerge as overburden, making them come to be horrible-tempered and ill. These kids aren't ruined. They just have diverse requirements. One method to assist them is to play track which gives an enhance to the clever element of the thoughts with the cause that the instinctive component is permitted to go with the drift. It allows them to experience more content material with themselves, organized to regulate to the movements and changes of their state of affairs all the more correctly and suddenly.

They mate soul-to-soul in choice to frame-to-body. Sexuality isn't a declaration of manliness or gentility, but rather the restriction of 1 human spirit to accomplice with some other spirit. Sexual expression is a fashion of correspondence so great, that intercourse with the surrender purpose of simply physical discharge is large to an Indigo. They pick out out their accomplices carefully, who opt for folks that instinctively recognize the profound otherworldly nature of the sexual exchange of power spoken to, through the sexual demonstration. Since an Indigo is recharged spiritually absolutely as certainly via way of each such revel in, they seem to have lower sex drives, locating that a top notch deal much much less but additionally interesting encounters are desirable over numerous easygoing encounters.

Intellectual skills or intellectual abilities of men and women bearing Indigo Aura

Their significantly superior highbrow alertness is one amongst the maximum great, however additionally the most traumatic problem of Indigos. They're vibrant and inquisitive, with intelligence that traditional intellectual tests can't diploma. Since those youngsters appear to be born expertise the whole lot, they're not inquiring for statistics besides for verification of the facts they already have.

It's as although they're trying out others to check whether or not they're honest or not.

Indigos have received large know-how of abstractions like time, distance, and space in their early a long time no longer because of the importance of these ideas for them, however because of their need for a deep statistics and verifying what they already understand. Because they get to the muse of factors, they're not fooled by the usage of the usage of appearances. When it's time for them to understand, they're going not to be delaying it.

The importance of education in the ones kids is wonderful. They're professional and unaffected with their proficiency, so any device that's insensitive to their dreams is demanding.

They want to be impartial, but no longer conceited; they will be in fact floating in with their very very own self. They have a deep choice for studying and upgrading their competencies. But they may't adapt to the normal getting to know pattern. Learning for them isn't unplanned. They study in a surrounding in which all statistics and understanding is mounted and referred. Subjects, subjects, and ideas can not exist in confinement for those children. They see the globe and thoughts as interconnecting portions of a larger organizational shape. They have an information of the way the quantities are going to healthy collectively. Indigo kids analyze top notch as soon as they will be recommended to comply with their very very own hobbies. They need a capacity for pursuing subjects deeply in place of glancing gently over the floor. They resent trainer-imposed alternatives on what and the manner they want to investigate. Indigos need to finish one region of have a take a look at in advance than transferring to the following idea, idea, or concept.

Their information takes area in Matrix patterns, conceptualizing the whole lot simultaneously. They see the general sample and each unit on the identical time. As a cease end result, they've got hassle explaining their mind and pics to others. Their education dreams are tremendous, and reading styles are great. They require schooling packages that may adapt to changes of their hobby; they need to understand concepts, and they want to be responsible for their international.

Once they'll be bored, annoyed, or intellectually underestimated, they typically withdraw into themselves and end up increasingly unwilling to make the efforts to remain concerned emotionally or mentally. Sometimes even throwing in the towel of school among a youngster and a mature being. They are not smug and don't keep in thoughts themselves brighter or more astute than their friends. They are looking for liberty, with a particular amount of guidance, to pursue their pastimes, and to fulfill theirs 'must recognize' spirit.

One need to recognize and cope with the Indigos' individuality. Indigos can't be pressured into doing some factor they don't want to do; they're not to honestly take delivery of something consequences that would get up. Indigos will remain cooperative as long as they're not befriended. They end up stubborn once they revel in positioned down and might cheerfully disrupt a whole classroom. To deal with Indigo youngsters, one need to supply them a breaker or intimation, in order that they're in a position to area a intellectual halt to their wondering technique.

Chapter 2: Emotional Engagement

Indigos are very clean about what they want. If one is giving them a desire, then one should better have the subjects to deliver. In case alternatives offered aren't introduced, that state of affairs threatens the credibility of that character in Indigo's life. They keep in mind guarantees. They can't in reality be fooled with the useful resource of such vague phrases as 'sooner or later' and 'quickly'. They need to realize precisely which 'at some point' or precisely how 'fast'. Without that means to nag, they will remind others of their guarantees, which they see as part of one's obligation to them. They do now not keep grudges or motel to emotional blackmail. They preserve in thoughts who can be relied on and who cannot. Indigos are not outspoken or overly friendly. They appear like self-contained. They are cautious with those to whom they supply their affection. While enormously content cloth and properly behaved, Indigos aren't spontaneous or brash. It is as even though they've seen all of it earlier than.

At many stages, Indigos in no way behave like youngsters. They appear extra mature than others of the same age, reacting with empathy and knowledge of lifestyles's little dramas. Indigo youngsters are greater self-contained than wonderful kids, wanting a whole lot less interplay with own family and pals. They do well if given good sized quantities of time on my own to pursue their personal pastimes and sports. They have active imaginations and regularly speak to themselves, misplaced in some other fact. They do well in environments that location easy and secure limits on their conduct on the equal time as no longer decreasing their want to find out and discover. Before which include an Indigo toddler inside the desire-making tool, adults want to kingdom the expectations, barriers, and goals. Indigos are short to cooperate at the same time as provided with simple alternatives, limits, and boundaries.

Few of the ordinary preliminary gaining knowledge of steps don't take a look at to Indigos, so dad and mom are frequently at a lack of what to do to manual, understand, and encourage the Indigo baby. These youngsters can't be emotionally bribed, nor can they be shamed into conforming to social standards and customs. Indigos will receive the repercussions of their conduct in choice to pass towards what they apprehend to be true. They can't be manipulated through guilt. The emotion of guilt is some factor that is not coming to them; they will be capable of't relate to it. Punishments like no food, or cutting down the privileges, are of no very last effects to an Indigo. Punishment even loses its cost if the man or woman in authority justifies it via pronouncing, "Do this because I say so."

Indigos ought to engage openly and spontaneously with only a few people. Early in their lives, they discover ways to be guarded and selective in sharing their thoughts, thoughts, and emotions. They bear in mind simplest slowly. Discarding the antique for the brand new is hard for them. They aren't the patron of a concept that 'extra moderen is typically higher'. They experience that on the same time as playing with an object or sporting a dress; they empower them with an detail of themselves, so throwing them away in reality to update them for a glowing one with out acknowledging the non-public essence instilled within the object, motives the deep emotional pains. If mother and father help them with good-bye rituals for the antique, whether or now not it is an historic and grubby filled animal or the circle of relatives vehicle, those kids may also moreover have an inherent experience of cycles and endings. To neglect about approximately this intuitive understanding is to defame one of the easy provides of those kids.

Indigo teenagers generally experience disconnected and out of sync with their associate company. Rebellious hairstyles, song, and garments look like a satire to them, a spoof of an alternate fact. Their experience of loneliness and isolation is similar to that experienced with the useful useful resource of a minority inside a set. In despair, they regularly retreat into a mist of drugs and alcohol in an attempt to disguise from loneliness in preference to make a rebellious lifestyle declaration. They recognize they do now not in form into the anticipated sample, and often they experience similar to the black sheep or the misfit of family, college, and society. Indigos, at a few deep diploma, recognize that we're all interrelated as a family, with out a dividing strains and no areas of possession or separation. Having a test those loss of differences, it isolates them in their knowingness.

Socio-way of life

The fantastic part of Indigos is that they may be sincere and sincere, so they may continuously say the truth, irrespective of how brutal it'll look to others. The recommendations of society do no longer advantageous them, and that they do what they experience is actual to them. They're no longer going to behave in a very unique manner in reality due to the fact an person guarantees them reputation as a prize. They don't recognize approximately guilt as they may be no longer doing something of their life to be appropriate. The cause in their life is to discover new strategies to permit absolutely everyone to specific themselves in a manner so that you can allow all to maintain to function as a worldwide.

They don't run away from troubles at the same time as human beings will anticipate. Instead, they are going to do things quietly and gracefully. The concept of being specific by no means motivates them as they perform a bit thing due to the truth they recognise that inside the returned of it there can be a moral rate connected to it and act therefore, as they price the relationships in which sharing and negotiations are required. But they'll not obey because of the creed. They can say no and suggest it; no quantity of prompting, suggesting, coaxing, praying, or punishing ought to cause them to change their minds.

They don't permit clearly everybody realise that they will be prying something painful or hard. They don't want human beings to experience sympathy for them. They tackle their troubles inside the only way regarded to them, and they don't want to consist of others in it. Since they may be very introverted, they'll be happy to do their non-public things on my own.

They are the individuals who look for a cushion of the family to experience extra steady. Thus whilst deciding on pals, Indigos favor to look for a person who may be their besties and companions on first after which be the fanatics. They pick out out someone based totally on their powerful character firmly rooted in truth.

Getting to realise them is a venture at the beginning, as they bypass again inner their shell whilst they are round people they are now not close to. They need someone they may consider; in any other case, they will be very guarded concerning their thoughts and feelings. In an intimate courting, they do now not need to have to display their conduct; therefore, they pick out friends who are sympathetic to their need to talk soul-to-soul, and to their unwillingness to comply. The tenderness and passionate engagement of the Indigo are the bonuses for individuals who are in a dating with them.

Finances and career alternatives

Indigos have a honestly poor information of cash. They see it as a element of the manipulative gadget employed thru a few human beings to modify and direct the movements and behaviors of others. Indigos will paintings because of the fact they experience the work. After all, it brings benefit and pride to themselves, and that they enjoy beneficial in doing it. If they locate the employment stupid or more work than they bargained for, they'll in reality give up.

To study Indigos acting on a challenge that pastimes them and absorbs their whole attention is to decide what courage really is. They in truth recognize what they require and what they do no longer want. This leaves Indigos with the complicated role of seeking to exercise session a way to protect themselves on the same time as doing what they experience. One in every of the techniques is for them to degree communally.

Living in a totally situation wherein they percentage costs and responsibilities works properly for them. Currently, Indigos discover exquisite delight running with their arms in occupations that need them to pay attention on the technique that's not intellectually stressful. Many of them have emerge as artisans, or perhaps repairmen.

They're practical, gentle-spoken, hardworking, and devoted personnel. They by using and big take jobs in such industries as improvement, and digital contracting, heating, and air-conditioning.

They are doing well in jobs that allow them resilience and flexibility however embody limits and hints, like inner control or constructing inspection. In the long term, as greater wishes and situations upward push up, Indigos will go with the flow in management positions because they want firsthand know-how received from revel in in repairing nowadays's technology. They'll understand what we need inside the future supported thru what we've within the present.

Spiritual Values

It is stated that very fewer human beings can absolutely understand the thoughts and emotions of a person with an Indigo Aura. Admirably conscious and expressed to be attuned to better planes, they act as bridges among this worldwide and additionally to the following. People who occur competencies like clairvoyance can also have an Indigo Aura. They relate this colour to the depths of inner intuition and a path of a extra reason. Indigo kids can effects recognize the complex spiritual requirements which can also moreover even fail the adults. They're believed to be beings of new power, coming for the primary time to hold inside the era of peace and concord. That is if the relaxation of the humans can learn how to pay attention to them.

Only an Indigo person can also actually thru way of final their eyes may be part of themselves with the lifestyles and universe round them. They're concept to own an innate connection to higher planes. This might also additionally flow from preceding lives or spiritual memories that humans have forgotten. It is said that human beings with an Indigo Aura regularly cross in non secular art work or be a part of a few spiritual ministries. They'll additionally discover themselves in an exceeding line of charitable paintings. Their propensity simply and connection to some thing extra drives them all through their lives to spread the maximum quantity of goodwill and knowledge as viable.

Indigos have a unique dating with the Higher Power. Most people go through in mind the higher being to be above us; our non secular evolution can be a manner of accomplishing and striving to raise ourselves through understanding, non secular practices, and examination of our personal internal selves. Indigos seem to very own an internal feel of the Higher Power. To them, the Higher Power may be a every day truth, no longer a theological concept as God is. Indigos can see that we are like an immature person, who're striving for spirituality, doing it with fear, now not with love. As they're born expertise the whole thing, they want quick get entry to to the general spectrum of what's identified in the paranormal or psychic international. As they may be aware that they recognize, they're plenty much less willing, as compared to others, to clear out or deny those change realities.

Spirituality, as expressed through an Indigo, is an example of what it method to live without the guilt and worry, commonly used by many faiths to intimidate and manipulate the masses. Indigos experience the person in their private divinity, that part of themselves as an correct copy of perfection. For them, their spirituality is a fact of being.

Knowing the entirety from shipping, it appears to return again again into this existence with all of the information of various instances, unique places, intact. It's as despite the fact that they maintain in mind in which they want to be before coming proper right here. This may be a end end result of spiritual evolution, or it may be an innate feature of the Indigo air of mystery people.

Indigos discover it clean to comply to institutionalized spiritual practices. Being children, they experience a reference to religious interests like meditation, and an appreciation of ceremonial accouterments like incense, remedy rocks, and smudge sticks. They frequently pick out them as playthings. They intuitively incorporate reverence and honor into their behavior, managing the religious devices passionately and with recognize. They respond easily and sincerely to prayers and meditation rituals; they seem to like their quiet time in addition to location. Indigos are spiritually eclectic, prepared to include many spiritual traditions, rituals, and image structures concurrently, taking peace and comfort from every. They're now not certain via vintage traditions, conduct, or notion systems.

These youngsters understand that there are order and pattern within the universe that has little to try to do with the rules and guidelines of different's form. They're prepared to convey together a holistic spirituality interior themselves, to make an inner temple able to accommodating plenty divergent perception systems.

Lavenders are one of these Aura colorings that have the capability for immoderate intuitive belief. They are progressive, touchy, artistically inclined, resourceful, channel divine strength, healer, visionary, or a spiritual instructor. For them, life is certainly a mystical global of journey full of illusions, visualizations, myths, and non secular beings. Lavenders aren't right right right here to shape a social declaration or trade the earth, or rescue others. They're right proper here to stimulate our imagination, to inspire our sense of wonder, and to keep the perception of magic alive in us. They are childlike, touchy, and innovative. Their innate capability to use their imagination makes them as a substitute innovative. They're additionally quite intuitive. Using facts, suited judgment, and motive, however, isn't clean for those gifted spirits. They are mild and unfastened spirits who aren't tremendous to have a look at any rules or being restricted with the useful resource of systems that dictate how they need to stay.

Their behavior frustrates others who need them to be robust and green. They do not apprehend what it approach to very very own a realistic undertaking or to build up coins. They are extra snug with great dimensions and imagined realities. They locate it tough to recognize the standards of time, vicinity, and physical depend. They experience events of their imaginations, but in reality, they can not gain some element robust.

They prefer to live of their illusionary international; They choose to spend their day experience of fact, in which existence is awesome and captivating. They live with the aid of their emotions and instinct, in preference to thru their mind. They require to be exempt from fact, to move in anything direction feels right at the time, and their hints exchange as regularly due to the fact the clouds do.

To stay on this 3-dimensional international is a notable project for Lavender people. For them, residing is easier in the dreamworld in desire to one which exists with the brand new technological tendencies. They can remodel their mind into works of artwork, thereby reinforcing the lives of others.

They have a separate manner to have a look at subjects; they see a transferring layer of shape, shape, and pattern, and people patterns shape a design, which lavenders dissolve and redecorate to create new structures and thoughts. To apprehend what lavenders are saying and to look what they're displaying, one ought so as to find out the shapes in clouds and divas inside the lawn.

They like the enterprise enterprise enterprise of folks that can see the functionality of their creativity and hovering ideas, and one which can form plans and take movement. They require very loving and affected person partners. If treated with softness and statistics, these loving Lavenders is probably friendly, responsive, enthusiastic, and devoted buddies. Partners can sooner or later find out the Lavenders' mind, innocence, and innovative imaginations charming and lovable.

Chapter 3: Lavender With Physical Reality

Lavenders are less bodily than unique shades; they pick to stay lifestyles in their goals and mind. For them, lifestyles is a mysterious global of adventure saturated with illusion, fascination, fantasies, imaginations, and religious beings. They bring with them an aura of fragility, and that they cope a lot much less well with the pressure of physical reality. They even appearance sick and mild. Because they don't take nourishment from nature. They like in-house sports, activities in a sheltered surroundings; they're no longer out of doors human beings, preferring to be internal, off from the modern-day sun and also the cold rain.

The fact of nature is hard for them to understand emotionally. Abstractly, they'll see the surprise in the earth, plants, bugs, and moreover the lifestyles cycle. But realistically, they discover that digging can be a grimy job, vegetation are the supply of stains and unpleasant odors on their arms, and bugs are repellent. They like a creative depiction of nature to the difficult reality of it. They seem to go along with the go with the flow via lifestyles; they'll be making equipped to step up and get the topics going, however in fact in no manner bothering to find out what's that which brings motivation in them to work.

Lavenders have a limited comprehension of the connection amongst time and region. They aren't inconsiderate, however the problem is that they may be struggling to modify to the variations in their myth life and real existence. They are permanently stuck of their dream global. To inform them to be attentive is to tug their interest from a dream global to this bodily world, regarding it's far a venture to lavenders.

To stress them to supply their interest and hobby to what is occurring in the present is to ask them to address truth. That is not awesome tough for a Lavender to do; it's miles painful, too. They experience that as though any person is pushing them once more into reality, the manner others experience on the equal time as someone isn't being allowed to sleep.

This shape of awakening is physiologically hard on the body's safety machine; in a greater excessive form, this technique has been used to torture struggle/political prisoners. When pals and circle of relatives grow to be too forceful, looking that Lavenders have to take responsibility, the Lavenders can become irritated and agitated. The simplest factor they need to is to stay a ways from fact; they handiest need by myself time with their snap shots and their goals.

Intellectual talents or highbrow capabilities of people bearing Lavender Aura

Lavenders one of the most talented Aura shades inside the manner of mentally retaining directly to the patters of progressive idea at the equal time as concurrently changing the numerous pieces to test particular viable outcomes. They can trade their interest detail, changing from the minute records to the general image. This is an remarkable exceptional, it absolutely is unrecognized in in recent times's realistic society. They percentage this capability to see patterns with one of a kind Personality Spectrums colors - Magenta and Green. Magentas examine the styles in 3-dimensional fact; they've got the potential to reduce and drape a sample on a dress form or to create an architect's scale model. Greens, however, see styles through time; they put together facts for clarity and general overall performance, developing timelines, flowcharts, and schedules, all even as not having seen the completed product.

Lavenders see a pattern through region. This way that once they have seen it in their thoughts's eye, they do not require reproducing it. In truth, their finest project is to preserve jogging till what they see in their head suits with what they might reproduce bodily. This enthusiasm to play with ideas, belief-workplace paintings, and psychic photos is the waft in their creativity. They are inclined to head past the ordinary limits of creativity, taking off new vistas of have a examine and explorations for the society to certainly take delivery of. Lavenders undergo the intuitive wondering techniques with recognize to the logical, systematic, intellectual thinking common to the Mental Auric Family sun sunglasses. They make a random database of the devices in the warehouse, and information of these products fill their mind.

As they live of their very non-public international of desires and fantasies, they'll be not restricted with the useful resource of constraints of time, location, materials, generation, or price range. To them, the whole lot is possible. So their every question starts offevolved with "why no longer?" Violets and Lavenders normally count on inside the same sample, but Lavenders don't placed any precondition immediately to themselves. For them, the enjoy of getting a dream or delusion is considerable. The toughest a part of the life of Lavender is to behave at the thoughts that generate of their minds. Lavenders must artwork enthusiastically to capture the choice-of-the-wisp; mind have to flourish and twist and redecorate them into this fact.

They are by using and huge seen. The photographs they get hold of, however, are having multisensory evaluations. So to explain them within the better shape, they strength their interest closer to describing the things coming to their minds through the usage of writing them down. As they interpret in their minds the answers to any trouble, it is transcribed into phrase images, wealthy with tonal, sensory texture. They have the terminology of the poet mixed with the warmth and devotion of an artist. Anything they will develop of their thoughts's eye is an possibility, even those matters which we do now not but have phrases to describe or provide an reason for.

Emotional engagement

If one is planning to be in a courting with Lavenders, they want to understand that lavenders are touchy, emotional, mischievous creatures, who are surely harmless and childlike - wonderful explorers of the imagination. Emotionally, they will be now not available for deeply committed relationships with others. Companions and kids need to apprehend that they'll express their love and caring casually. When they may be confident that they are not going to be dragged inside the every day chaos of physical existence, they will begin connecting but cannot precise it the identical manner others need. They don't need to get concerned in every day humdrum sports activities of everyday lifestyles, as to them those are the maximum tedious and uninteresting hobby and can lead them to break out into their non-public heads for emotional and intellectual restoration.

They have hassle making and maintaining deep tiers of human interaction. They preserve a part of themselves constantly in reserve, unavailable to precise people for near, heat interplay. Ultimately, to emerge as entangled in the complexities of a dating could require that Lavenders surrender that part of themselves that needs the freedom to discover the outer limits of their fantasies and their creativity.

Lavenders are born with a energetic imagination and with the energy to form new and one-of-a-type realities; if no longer always practical, they're constantly exciting, presenting meals for idea for others. They're the least grounded of all the colours. They stay in their non-public realm of goals and fantasies. It appeared that they came into this fact after retaining aside from a few detail that could supply shape or choice to their lives. They face troubles in growing and preserving a gadget of values and ideals, and moreover regularly adopting the tips of various more potent personalities as their personal. They endure existence as despite the fact that they don't truely belong, as though they don't in shape in. They discover it difficult to call any region as their home. They feel out of sync and have a tendency to shield themselves in the lower back of an opaque veil. When encountered through way of way of others who need a few facts, Lavenders regularly fall again right right into a big-eyed innocence that pronounces, "Are you asking me?"

Lavenders are the dreamers of the spectrum, and they experience all varieties of self-induced altered states of hobby. They continuously daydream, on occasion drifting away within the middle of a sentence, steady within the movement they see of their minds. The terms we are announcing can flip a transfer inner their mind, discharging a drift of inner photos. We on the floor are unaware of what's going on inner them. But, for them, what's going on inner their thoughts is so wealthy that outside truth seems

superfluous.

In our society nowadays, a outstanding emphasis is being given on traumatic and nurturing, Lavenders as a determine discover it difficult to conform to the function of loving, traumatic, and nurturing accomplice and determine. They do all they need to do, but they are capable of't deliver in assessment to others. They can see and are privy to what they want to do, but in reality, they'll be no longer in a position to relate to it. These versions begin constructing up a feeling of guilt. Lavenders who can not balance their innate nature with their revel in of guilt generally withdraw internal themselves emotionally and physical.

Socio-manner of existence

Socially, Lavenders are loners, and they may be scared that others will now not apprehend their style of living. They spend most of their time with their thoughts and thoughts. They are the unfastened spirits who don't want to make certain thru policies and duties. They are very sensitive and childlike. They are happy to have a partner who can offer them with guide, admire their modern paintings, and manipulate all of the monetary topics and exceptional regular obligations. They never particular their feelings, or what's going indoors their mind as they've got a worry of being criticized. Fighting the concern from time to time they adapt as an entire lot as a tool wherein they masquerade as they're conforming, but simply, their mind is one million miles away. They best want recognize for the revolutionary stature in their paintings. They are disciplined in working on their thoughts, however they do not perform a little thing to make a social declaration. They art work due to the truth something has popped up of their mind.

In a relationship in which they experience emotionally and physical ordinary, Lavenders are revolutionary, imaginative, bold, and experimental, willing to be engaged physical just so their minds are unengaged to roam the astral airwaves. It's as although Lavenders slip out of this truth whilst sexual love, understanding that their accomplice and their very personal our our bodies will remind them to head back.

Lavenders have loose ties with their households and a few near buddies. Of all of the aura colours, they will be folks who require the least quantity of attention for the bodily and emotional nurturing provided by those relationships. Instead, they pick out solitude with time for daydreaming. They turn out to be actively worried with their intellectual lives; their creations, writings, or unique varieties of creative expression have an entire existence in their very very personal. These creations are basically each relation to them.

Sexual expression is one region wherein Lavenders can keep on on this international what they locate within the dream. They're a number of the important sexually progressive, the most inclined to test, of all the Personality Spectrums colorations. Be that as it is able to, Lavenders do put confines on sexual exploration beyond which they obtained't tour. These constraints depend on their requirement for emotional and psychic properly being. Their policies and boundaries are deliberate, and their highbrow and bodily well being is aware of that doesn't in reality follow the regulations of an explicitly hindered society.

Chapter 4: Finances And Profession Options

Although Lavenders are first-rate and excellent beings, close to working, they favor to paintings in quiet, low-pressure environments that allow them ok quantity of time to go of their dreamland and connect with their imagination beings. Regular going for walks hour's process is painful for them due to the truth they may be required to place masses of intellectual interest.

Neither are they correct at calculating or analyzing information, nor you may although anticipate them to prepare something as they may be too forgetful and scattered. They honestly have issues getting their customers' orders in retailers. They do artwork at their very very own pace; they might't be rushed or pressured.

When it consists of coins, they may be just like a child; they want very little concept of coins as a motivation, a medium of alternate, or a yardstick for measuring fulfillment. Once they've got it, they may spend it, and if they don't have it, they don't. For them, coins is form of a exercise. One who wins includes all the cash. However, they frequently get bored and mentally estrange from the game earlier than the stop give up result has been determined, leaving the alternative gamers with a hollow victory. Lavenders aren't quitters; they truely depart.

They can do nicely within the fields of performing arts, and theater, because of the fact over here they may get the threat to find out their imagination and creativity. Occupations which are appealing to Lavenders encompass the following: Storyteller, Dancer, Set Designer, Actor, HouseDdecorator, Clothes fashion designer, Mime artist, Teacher, Educator, Artist (especially fable art), Writer (particularly kids's books).

Spiritual Values

Lavenders have outstanding capability for religious increase. They need the threat to find out the Higher Being of their personal unique manner and time. They are loose birds, and that they don't bind themselves to a person set of perception systems. They need unfastened get proper of entry to to recognize any concept or notion that attracts them. GOD to them is a amazing idea to investigate, however if a few element attempts to bind them to pointers and responsibilities, they opt to go away that area. Personal freedom appeals to the ones human beings. In their quest to search for Spiritual companies lavenders flip every table round - they be a part of ashrams, Chant mantras, and spend severa energy - but as each machine is certain to 3 underlying perception system, it will become tough, beyond lavenders' scope to comply to.

Their inherent nature motives them to be associated with their spirit publications all of the greater productively; however, it could damage their running lives. This is due to the fact they may alternatively no longer harm down things, liking to go with their gut instincts.

Crystal is one of the rarest visible sunglasses as an air of mystery colour. Individuals with crystal colour are the maximum accommodating of all the different air of thriller color humans and can be visible as a real duplicate of the individual they're assembly with. They display each horrific and high-quality functions of each folks; they may be surely defensive themselves via emotional camouflage and in turn, they assimilate with exclusive air of mystery colorings much like chameleons do. When they're in sync with their energies, they get alongside quite nicely with nearly everyone. However, generally people get stressed via their inconsistencies, because the greater they may be meeting humans, the more they're soaking up, and the more they may be soaking up, the extra their personalities trade.

Crystal children are a few other specific beauty of humans. In a global limited and troubled thru a materialistic mind-set, they will be said to comply with their hearts as idealists.

As the color of Aura is the individual of the coloration, they constantly take in electricity from the whole thing and all of us round them, and so they're the clearest and purest varieties of energy healers available to humankind. They are able to being a conduit or channel for recuperation energy. Being herbal healers; the Crystals' gift is to assist humans around them to smooth blockages from their minds and souls, and to permit the natural healing technique to start for them. Not all and sundry they'll be assembly is prepared or prepared for this energy shift, and they will experience an power drain in the presence of Crystal Aura humans.

It is difficult for them to apprehend this present with them, and that is the maximum crucial project for them. At instances they get confused or disturbing by means of the usage of the ones energies. They resonate at a higher frequency which makes them over sensitive, touchy and fragile, because of which they avoid businesses and gatherings and prefer to be by myself.

Interaction of crystals with Physical Reality

Crystal people sense separated from the bodily international, and because of this they're obsessive approximately their private area. They are the human beings obsessed with cleanliness and neatness, and it's miles hard for them to test some detail that is unpleasant, dirty, or unattractive. In the choice to create an appropriate picture of the location having untouched palaces, which they have got of their thoughts, however while in reality they will be able to't discover that, they revel in horrified. To them, this physical surroundings is harsh, unfriendly, and cold.

They are very touchy to noise and different kinds of pollutants. They are very touchy beings and can without troubles get shattered as their our bodies are very fragile. Health is continuously a place of scenario for them. Almost something can move incorrect with Crystals. As they are proficient with strength assimilation, they may even take at the health troubles of their partners. They vibrate at very excessive frequency, and being sensitive and inclined they must spend time in solitude and quiet meditation, to easy any horrible energy impacts that they may have absorbed. They experience uncomfortable in massive organization gatherings and like to be by myself, in order that they most effective permit a few close to friends and family people to visit them that too for brief durations of time.

They like to paintings and play with soil; it now not exceptional satisfies them however additionally offers a sense of stability. They sense emotionally higher when they spend time of their garden - going for walks with vegetation, or growing and drying herbs. It offers them no longer satisfactory the emotional delight, but additionally presents them with an abundance of serene time on my own with God and nature - an crucial for their suitable highbrow, spiritual, physical, and emotional balance.

They aren't capable of visualize what they want, as at the same time as interacting with a person. They stay with their energies and unknowingly chameleonize themselves, to be a one-of-a-type character; and forgetting that they are a selected individual and their desires are unique.

Intellectual abilities or highbrow talents of people bearing Crystal Aura.

Crystals are very sensible. They want to look at a large variety of subjects and characteristic a mastery of obtained and intuitive records. To achieve their better desires, most of the crystals advantage a couple of stages. They invest lots of time considering what they accept as true with in., meditating and praying over the facts in their lifestyles.

They are very spiritual, as they artwork through the crown chakra, however very few are able to realise this. For them, real spirituality has stress and authority. Those crystal individuals who are not able to recognize this fact approximately themselves are not in a position to connect to the better beings in a deep custom designed connection. This is their inner motivation, and in the occasion that they leave out this, their existence motive receives lacking. Their lifestyles is then without a doubt disadvantaged of God's love and flows as emotionally charged unresolved circulate, with out a sympathy.

They are avid readers, researchers, and commonly hardworking, accountable, and diligent. But it's far hard for them to offer interest and efforts to the subjects which require them to rote. So the subjects like that of maths, remote places languages, accounting are few to say which they haven't any interest in. Whereas, they're quite precise and supply their great inside the fields of indoors designing and completed creativity.

They are natural healers, having an inborn ability to heal the encircling people, so they excel within the healing arts-medication, psychotherapy, nursing, massage, or pores and skin. Crystals may be part of their herbal abilties to the intuitive way they have got a have a look at. They are bright, short, and psychologically active. They observe society via TV, theater, and movies, and this getting to know is vital for them as this makes them aware about the conduct, that one wishes to be as part of society.

They withdraw into paintings, books, and /or meditation, so that they keep away from coping with relationships, chaos, or an excessive amount of noise. They pick out out books that provide them an notion into the behavior and ethics of present day-day society. They additionally opt to look at inspirational books. They keep away from reading literature.

Emotional engagement

Emotionally, Crystals can show as lots as be aloof, faraway, and rigid. They react as though they may be following a pattern rehearsed or taught to them; in region of spontaneous motion to conditions, it looks like they agree to a script. They are shy personalities, and they keep themselves in the historical past. Not because they will't perform but simply hiding because of their disability to react spontaneously. They rarely show their deepest feelings. In disaster too, they select doing the proper subjects in preference to their spontaneous moves. They have a deep-rooted fear that their proper emotions may be misunderstood, and they'll be therefore are reluctant to percentage those deep additives of themselves.

They can soak up and refract unique sun shades; the quantity of impact of other air of mystery colorings is proportionate to the interaction over a period. For instance, a few additives of Crystal's air of secrecy will replicate like that of inexperienced at the same time as they interact with a Green. They camouflage their personality by way of soaking up rays of diverse air of thriller hues. In doing so, Crystals furthermore take at the tendencies and eccentricities, fashion, and mind of the alternative sunglasses. People round them aren't able to understand their conduct, and it brings communication breakdowns. Parents confront Crystal children who're inconsistent in their subject and regulations. Parents also are confused thru way of these kids as they retreat emotionally, giving no clue as to what they're thinking or feeling. Parents do now not comprehend how to hook up with the ones youngsters on a everyday diploma. As they appear so sensitive and fragile, other greater Physical Family Colors wants to non-public them. Yet their inclination stays towards GOD. They experience that God handiest can recognize them; else all others don't. They are searching out approval from humans very near them, they even search for tips at the manner to react in social gatherings, and that they become genuinely relying on others to deal with the outer international.

They commonly bypass inwards and isolate themself in the instances of pressure, which indicates their emotional unavailability or say air of secrecy of coldness. Emotionally, they will be very fragile. They resonate with excessive-frequency energies masses simply so their concerned structures are constantly getting ready to overload. They see the excellent strong vicinity to shield themselves is to transport inwards when they withdraw; they leave others trying to wager what took place. They pick to be by myself, no longer due to any highbrow trauma, however just they need to be left with their inner self. This reference to inner self proves to be useful for them in their restoration sports activities activities, in which they will be capable of use their middle strength with out simple thru private emotional involvement.

Socio-way of life

Being social is one of the hardest regions of lifestyles for Crystal Aura People and for others to be with them. They are shy in nature, and wanted self-assurance, and mixed with each the ones attributes; they lack self notion in social gatherings. Thus they prefer to be withdrawn, reserved, and be by myself. They enjoy that they do not apprehend the way to behave socially; all they do on this manner is that they studies from severa property, like family, pals, television, and movies. They can also grow to be hypercritical of themselves and others, hurting their already low feel of conceitedness. They usually enjoy uneasy in a large crowd, and they end up with out issue disoriented and compelled in social situations.

As their coping mechanism is limited, they positioned the duty of the entirety going on on others. They even research from the environment which surrounds; their verbal exchange uses pretty some fillers terms like 'need to' and 'ought'. They apprehend life as an onstage drama without scripts, and they'll be now not easy about what others are expecting from them.

They opt to be by myself, as any interest which requires them to engage intensively with everybody repels them, and intercourse is the same for them as it requires them to co-mingle their charisma with others, which they take as a danger to their individuality. The after-results of intercourse are too excessive physical in addition to emotionally on them, that they decide upon celibacy as it brings peace and the possibility to song their lives to their individual herbal clocks.

Finances and career alternatives

Crystals are very responsible and careful with their cash. They are law-abiding people; they may't even agree with approximately breaking/bending laws, in order that they make sure to pay all their dues on time. For Crystals, to lose their freedom, to be placed below scrutiny is disgraceful. They are quick to recognize the situations and are able to observe and make their solid and realistic alternatives rapid. They don't go for creativity and prefer to do vintage school organization shape of, with the resource of using making an funding in actual property or coping with an gift enterprise.

They are not suited at installing any new commercial enterprise corporation setup; neither they could deal with it with out anyone's assist. They don't opt to art work with new agencies, however select an aged corporation residence. Wealth and investments are too particular, too actual, for a Crystal to cope with and no longer using a problem.

They are herbal healers; that is one in each in their herbal developments and the high-quality of traits of Crystal Aura peoples in case you need to do properly in enterprise associated with the properly-being of humanity. They do nicely in jobs concerning the restoration segment from being a scientific medical doctor's receptionist to being a physician.

They can keep themselves distant, aloof with their customers as they sense that they have got been referred to as to heal, now not to entertain. The place wherein they may be capable of do properly is, wherein they may receive the possibility to do duties in which they may be able to upload their rate. They need an organized, non violent environment and a everyday. They are proper to move for any administrative center or art work state of affairs that requires repetition and attention to detail.

They are an amazing Spiritual Master trainer (no longer public university structures), as they'll lightly guide others at the direction of deeper have a examine and understandings.

Chapter 5: Spiritual Values

Crystal Aura color individuals are a rare mixture of intelligence and spirituality; they will be interested in God via highbrow evaluation, studies, and exercising, or they may pursue higher degrees of spirituality thru soul searching practices and deep meditations. Sometimes, they're capable of have interaction in each. Their closing cause is to acquire internal peace and divine stillness. They need to discover answers to all of the non secular queries so that you can offer them with the notice of who God without a doubt is and the manner they will be associated with God.

For them, spirituality manner dwelling a existence of stillness that comes from learning that eventually soon, they may be going to be one with their right being. Crystals are a completely precise, delicate, and fragile coloration humans with their private spiritual mechanism to attach and align with the healing energies available.

When they accomplice with their existence's paintings, they are energetic, glad, simply functioning, and at peace with themselves and others round them. However, after they can not well known their gift and work with it, their lives are depressed, poor, difficult, and complete of melancholy. They emerge as lonely and silly as even though they may be surviving, pleasant till they may be able to vanish.

They vibrate on a excessive frequency of the religious realm, which makes them extra fragile and sensitive; however, it increases the capability of facts others and allows them gain healings of their our bodies. They have a psyche of the purest spiritual form, able to managing pinnacle levels of religious vibrations. They take this as a gift and make this as their existence's motive. Assimilating knowledge from severa resources and then facts and arranging them to settle in their intellectual database takes them to spend masses of time. It moreover calls for them to stay in a quiet and calm environment, a long way from the confusion of the area.

Black is a paranormal colour associated with fear and the unexplained (black holes). Black denotes splendor, ritual, demise, evil, sadness, mourning, and mystery. It absorbs every lightwave and displays now not whatever, so it brings hundreds of distress and restlessness with itself. Black offers the have an effect on of belief and depth, however a black background diminishes readability. A black get dressed could make you look thinner. It is regularly used with a terrible significance (blacklist, black humor, 'black lack of life'). Black denotes strength and authority. In heraldry, black is the photograph of grief.

Similarly, the Black air of mystery is one the severa few auras which may be considered as typically awful. It's now not critical that an character who's carrying a Black air of mystery is inaccurate or an unpleasant person. It's a fable and has been found to be incorrect, in a huge wide form of instances.

Anyone may have Black air of thriller relying on their physical, intellectual, or emotional health. Black strength is carefully related to as a minimum one's health. It can represent a few fitness troubles that one isn't aware of. Or it may additionally display extraordinary fitness problems one is aware about approximately but isn't always prepared to simply accept and cope with. Being in rebuttal is severe, and your aura is right here to warn you of that. The coloration of charisma modifications to black if those healths problems begin developing below your pores and pores and skin. You can also moreover moreover begin feeling as something is off internal your self, but it's difficult to definitely acquire or perhaps bear in mind that it could be some thing vital.

The first reason in the back of a black air of secrecy is that the unwillingness to forgive self or others.

These human beings must discern out the cause and want to forgive the man or woman and take delivery of the apology that is required to manoeuvre on and go through the horrible feelings which is probably causing the black aura to be seen. Black in the air of mystery isn't always locked to unique mistakes and as an alternative emanates from one's frame on the same time as the focal point and energies don't seem to be in sync and are imbalanced in determine upon of ache or uncooked negativity.

This may be now not the simplest purpose, however it's one the numerous numerous reasons prolonged contamination can be an detail in a single's black air of mystery. A black air of mystery implies problems from a number of the person's beyond existence and hurts which might be affecting their gift life and thinking. It moreover illustrates the concern of narrowing one's capability to convert terrible energies.

The extra you circulate toward immoderate first-rate electricity, the colour of your air of thriller can even begin to exchange. There are many factors which have an effect at the shade of an charisma – those are in particular your emotions, thoughts-set, mind, individual, and physical state of affairs.

Black is the shade of Vaccum or hollowness. There are numerous one-of-a-kind strategies that vacuum can specific itself, however human beings with black auras always locate themselves laid low with acute, unexplainable despair. They normally fill their alone time with some form of leisure; you received't discover black aura human beings playing quiet-non violent by myself time. Whenever they may be going to spend time by means of themselves, they'll do it with some hobby or hobby to preserve their thoughts occupied. Usually, when a black charisma spends loads of time by myself in quiet meditation, it's because they had been overcome with the aid of way of a experience of pain and find out it difficult to do some element in any respect. Black auras are tortured souls.

They deliver deep-rooted lack of confidence, and to mask this up; they want to hold a function of power and status. They are unbiased, sturdy-willed, and decided, with a display of grace and refinement that indicates that they're constantly on top of things of any situation. Somewhere this is right, as they want to hold their emotions hidden from others. They want to hold others at a distance from them so no one can come round them and they are blanketed from the negativity of others.

They aren't proper at sharing their emotions and emotions; consequently, they preserve things deep indoors them. They are very methodical, ensuring they complete the whole lot as required right all the manner right down to the maximum minute detail. If they aren't careful, they're grabbing for strength to cover their non-public troubles could make them power-hungry without them absolutely expertise why.

Interaction of Black with Physical Reality

Black isn't always a eternal Aura color; it is genuinely protecting one's air of mystery at the prevailing time. If we say in less tough phrases, a symptom in place of a surrender cease end result. Auras radiate energy outwards, on the same time as the horrible ones draw strength into themselves, sucking subjects in like a black hollow and making someone like Energy-Vampire. Having a Black Aura way that over a time body, your moves, emotions, and different factors strolling have someplace suppressed your proper self. And to combat once more to the world one has modified himself and strolling in a way appears great to him, this is taking him far from the soul reason. The darkness consumes the mild of want, growing hopelessness and trapping and suppressing your natural air of mystery. It is not your identity, not the 'actual' you, and it will exceptional stand round so long as you allow it.

Those with Black Aura are self-inspired and determined. This requires them to take complete authority for themselves. They must recognize and recall precisely what they want and take the desired steps to gather it. In doing this, they will be capable of benefit peace and revel in more emotionally focused.

Although bodily exercising is extraordinary for them, human beings with a Black Aura aren't inquisitive about bodily hobby for the sake of it. They don't need to play for the fun's sake; they need a reason at the back of it.

Remember that black auras are viable for quick phrases throughout times of grief, severe pressure, and splendid emotional or highbrow troubles. They may be remedied evidently as the unhappy factors lose their grip on them or one recover from grief with time. In case a person involves apprehend that he has a Black Aura he can take the next steps, following the strategies to rectify it.

Intellectual abilties or intellectual skills of ladies and men bearing Black Aura

Black as they absorb all energies from the surroundings into them, they may be exceedingly intuitive, and their understanding is secret. They are completely unpredictable, and it's miles hard to decide their next go along with the float or motion. They increase properly of the employer as they've got a command on their conversation; they're hard personnel, and right at strategic choice making. They are social beings and do properly in the region of advertising and marketing and advertising.

They want to be in a energy function. They like to be very methodical, and make certain that they have got followed each minute element in doing any technique. They need to be greater cautious; otherwise, their gaining strength to cover themselves can also turn up into a few different extreme problem.

Emotional engagement:

A Black Aura is frequently consultant of transformation - one is both coping with stress and grief or is in a country of emotional disturbance. Either way, this isn't always one's place to be and isn't always their eventual tour spot. Life does now not stop proper right here. Those who need to change and make a comeback can constantly do that and get themselves out from this shady air of mystery realm.

Sometimes, one is going into grief due to their courting and starts accumulating dark energies, and looking for negativity in every detail, and make this negativity as a part of them. One may be feeling lonely or depressed because of long-distance relationships or is managing a number of an unresolved combat. The persistent loss of courting also can motive a darkening air of mystery. If one has been via a breakup, this can cause quite a few emotional misery. If one is unmarried for a long term and no longer been fortunate in their search for companions and surrendered to the inflicting depression and begins offevolved feeling like they are now not going to locate someone, the Black Aura can appear.

When one starts feeling like this for their love life, it is for high pleasant that they'll be having an underlying trouble that wants to be resolved. This is something one need to cope with inside them in advance than you pursue any similarly relationships.

Socio-lifestyle

Socially, people with Black Aura are related to luxurious, wealth, and plenty of cash. They regularly lead a flowery, expensive lifestyle and need plenty of coins to sense fulfilled. Their social recognition and recognition are critical to them.

These matters can come from the darkness and inclined element internal them that has delivered about the Black Aura in the first region.

While in the united states of america that has added approximately a Black Aura, they war to peer all people as equals. They have a tendency to provide choice to people who are a part of their international and might in shape their reputation.

This will motive them to miss out on a whole lot of deep, great friendships with great individuals who definitely don't have some of money.

Chapter 6: Finances And Career Options

People with Black Aura are electricity-pushed people; they want the electricity to create a gap just so no character can approach them. They actually have a agency perception that everyone has the right to stay in prosperity and abundance. They don't similar to the segmentation of wealthy and terrible. They moreover assume each person want to get the identical possibility to expose themselves, and all people has to art work difficult.

They are ambitious, tough-operating, and inclined to do a little detail to fulfill their desires. They are self-stimulated spirits, and those dispositions of them take them to heights in some detail they do and cause them to a success.

They are aware of a manner to unfold their enterprise business enterprise, and they use all the ones approaches to unfold their employer. They go to social activities to create a community. They select out to offer and acquire recommendation associated with wealth and different factors beneficial to all people.

People with Black Aura are a a achievement enterprise company proprietor or defensive up a few better authority figures primarily based mostly on their highbrow functionality, willpower, and conversation skills. They are having great management abilities too, and typically have a tendency to govern agencies, managing tasks and sports.

They hold prominent positions within the society, or corporations they paintings for - wherein they'll want to make important selections and control others. They are enthusiastic about their career and are an normal workaholic. They decide upon jobs that require extended hours and difficult paintings.

There preferred professions are of being a banker, attorney, flesh presser, market specialists, and producers.

Spiritual Values

Spiritually they'll be pretty improved souls, and they take their spirituality in trying to find energy from the better self. Sometimes being ego-driven, they trust themselves to be equal to GOD. They get worried within the awful sides of spirituality and connect with the Left-Hand group.

They revel in the use of their reference to the Higher beings for the attainment of energy and on occasion even venture or fight with the divine forces. With their excessive will power and their ego and mindset of going to any extent to matters they need to achieve, they do the inflexible meditations and gain the powers which can be tough for ordinary humans.

They get majorly concerned in Tantric Kriyas, Witchcraft, Black Magic, and other such sciences.

White is one of the maximum magical colorings! It is one of the rarest shades to have a take a look at in the Aura spectrum. Bearing a white air of mystery is the most magnificent occurrence. White is the shade of purity, honesty, truthfulness, and a country of attention. This manner that any character with a white charisma will replicate the ones objects as a part of their character and conduct.

White is the color of enlightened spirits; it suggests that the individual has been illuminated to the whole lot on this international that is right, suitable, nice, and high-quality. It symbolizes an awoke awareness and an growth in higher dimensions. A white aura may additionally mean someone is receptive to possibilities to start off all all over again. They personal endless capability.

White auras constitute a kingdom of absolute purity of an character radiating from the within. This aura in itself is the most resistant of auras to any form of horrific energies that commonly surround us. Like all auras, there's a herbal shade of tints associated with this shade, beginning from the purest white to the worrisome cloudy or murky tones.

White Aura also can supply meanings. It can also mean every a Beginning or Destination. Beginning happens with shipping. In Infants, it's far been discovered that they bring about a white air of secrecy. This suggests their untainted and innocent kingdom organized to be molded through life's feelings and evaluations. Adults can also possess white auras, and that they do. Particularly dad and mom which can be with strong spiritual connections. Irrespective of the origins, there may be regularly no doubt that a White Aura represents real and unselfish goodness.

While people with white light are commonly rare, now not all white air of mystery's are the identical. The colorations, energies, and solar sunglasses can range from man or woman to man or woman, and each technique a few element marginally one-of-a-kind.

Pure white includes an detail of truce and settling. Many undergo in mind that God's non-public moderate is powerful and white – this illustrates the energy and splendor of a White Aura in someone. The herbal white colour can assist every bodily and non secular restoration further to take away horrible energies.

Within the arena of pure white, there are typically organizations. The first one includes toddlers, newborns, and more youthful kids. These are those who are new on the earth, and characteristic little or no revel in of the worldly affairs and are although ignorant in mind, body, and soul. They are untouched souls and haven't nonetheless made any reason-pushed efforts to gain this colour or its energies. The subsequent company consists of human beings who've obtained information with their developing age, and now they have got have become older. They are those who've seen each element of life, been through usaand downs of life, and feature labored difficult the whole time to reap religious enlightenment. They can be someone who's significantly non secular and has decided their practices strictly or a person who is without a doubt religious and has worked very difficult to forge a moral path of their existence. It is uncommon for adults to benefit this coloration, and it's a few element that is typically extra cautiously related to angels.

The 2d group within the picture is of non-pure white. This is a hard and fast of those folks that are wearing a white charisma, but because of some linked tones or solar sunglasses in them, they may be non-natural white. The auras and energies they invent are nevertheless that of white, and they however represent similar topics, but they have got a dark tone to them. These solar sunglasses can vary some problem amongst slightly off-white coloration to almost completely grey. This darkish colour represents energies which is probably weighing one down.

These human beings are having brilliant trends of white air of thriller, but have a few aspect indoors them this is imperfect and tainting their lifestyles and happiness. Most in all likelihood, weight is non secular. It can be possible that sure doubts are there which one can't get happy or some of their choice which they are forcefully leaving as it may impede one's spiritual progress. It can also simply be the truth that one has come from plenty of struggles in his life and now want time to nurture and find out his spirituality.

It isn't impossible, but a tedious undertaking for non-herbal white air of thriller humans to gain the purest vibrant stage. They want to decide out the motive for the impediment and need to achieve this in competition to that and remove it. This can also require them to take a holiday or using a few precise technique to interrupt out their each day flow deep in self for introspection temporarily.

Interaction of White with Physical Reality

As maximum of the human beings in the pure White Aura are toddlers, younger kids, and newborns, so they'll be absolutely in their private world grasping and searching on the happenings around. They are effective to the grooming of the society and the energies; they are certainly reflecting the same into the surroundings. They are not energetic game enthusiasts on this diploma but simply act as an observer.

Adults with herbal white notable light are in phrases with their spirituality, and they'll be in this form of thrilled and contended degree that they'll be beyond the physicality. They experience the need to spread facts, to heal, for the properly-being of society. Like a wanderer, they promote and spread pleasure and happiness to all spherical.

People with non-exquisite herbal air of mystery, are someplace stuck in each day lifestyles's sports activities and are suffering for resolution with that to obtain their spirituality.

Chapter 7: Highbrow Capabilities Of Humans Bearing White Aura

A easy white air of secrecy is a illustration of the purity of thoughts, and additionally the individual bearing them isn't always stimulated by way of the use of muddied thoughts or negative emotions. As missing this readability, the frame lacks the degree of stability.

With their loyal thoughts-set, their workmates can depend on them as soon because the case gets tough. They're inclined to cope with greater art work inside the occasion that they want the time and strength.

Unfortunately, they'll now and again go overboard as quickly as they're trying and please human beings. This doesn't constantly advocate that they're sucking up. This is frequently just their authentic purpose to provide the wonderful pleasant of help to others.

Sometimes, people with white air of mystery can lack objectives. This is frequently due to the fact they opt to try to do the hard and difficult paintings.

Therefore, maximum of them will reject the marketing in particular if this can save you them from doing the objects that they love.

It isn't going for the White humans to provide an motive at the back of delays or troubles in the place of work. This makes them extremely dependable.

However, they're going to nonetheless prioritize helping others over their artwork. They can sacrifice some thing, collectively with their work for the greater unique. Nonetheless, they're going to do that with out a signs of regret.

The power that's being launched with the aid of human beings with White Aura is pure, and that could repel unwell intentions and evil energies. While they do not have the sensitivity of individuals with a Purple

Aura, however they stand for every non secular recognition and additionally the willingness to help parents which might be struggling.

When starting a commercial agency challenge or following a emblem, or choosing an alternative career route, those who radiate a White Aura will continuously be lucky. They do not really repel awful energies in addition they entice prosperity and achievement. Their industrial company can be effective for the motive that they may remodel a preferred detail into some factor

Socio-way of life

Due to your heightened spirituality and sensitivity, you'll be greater reserved and introverted. There are few humans whom one will need to bring in sync with one's personal time, as they're going to empty your energy. Observe how people make you enjoy and offer some time therefore.

Having white strength way you're aware about the desires and feelings of others. Not simplest are you capable of help your self in complicated or overwhelming conditions, however you furthermore can also assist others inside the equal way. Those in want are attracted to you and are searching out for recommendation because of the reality they understand you'll be able to assist them. You'll revel in deep and loving relationships packed with loyalty and useful resource. You're also able to heal others via your first-rate power which wards off the lousy just through manner of manner of

being there.

Emotional engagement

Those with white aura can growth friendships with out troubles, as long as the man or woman holds their moral views and is a type person. As friends, they're fiercely unswerving and might usually be willing to assist -

sort of parent. The drawback to those relationships is that human beings with plenty of flaws or insecurities may additionally enjoy judged and unworthy. Those gifted with this air of secrecy don't do that for a cause; it really takes region, way to their natural nature and connection to the subsequent electricity that drives them to positives.

Unlike the blue, pink, and violet auras with regards to a romantic relationship, and finding a associate, companions of those with a white air of thriller have to analyze the dangers. Their purity and innocence make them gullible - this will be a few aspect you want to be cautious about and help them apprehend. Reciprocally for this greater strive and mindfulness, they're going to accumulate the inner most, maximum excessive degree of love they've ever professional. However, it's essential to be aware that you actually acquired't be their entire international. They want an innate preference to assist and serve others, and this may be a assignment to them but. If you get within the manner of this part of them, they may now not need to be within the dating.

Finances and profession alternatives

Money is one of these things which doesn't depend to them, and they may be glad in a administrative center this is social and gives interactions with others around. They want to spend their lifestyles in supporting and reaping benefits others. If their profession isn't always on the route and any of those matters is lacking, they may find it difficult to prevail as they might with out hassle get distracted. Common career paths for a person with a white aura embody nurses, therapists, and animal rescues, some issue wherein they may use their particular studies and help the radiance glow can shine. They are not the hassle creators. In truth, they'll be able to deliver harmony in the place of business. They are in particular dependable, social, and dependable assets.

That stated, assisting a person is more than a few thing to them, and it is not remarkable for a White to surrender his or her hobby for that one super deed. Even in the ones times, there are genuinely no apologizes, and it's miles continuously nicely-intentioned.

White air of mystery usually emanates purity, and whilst there is purity, there may be no space for negativity inside the surroundings, it moreover benefits them who're close to them with their presence. While they will be now not having that hypersensitivity of violets, they will be in no way less non secular and decided of their energy to help those suffering and are in need.

Those who possess a white air of thriller make first rate friends and eternal partners, however their first name will continuously closer to their divine and unselfish calling to assist lives. This unique innocence of them comes at a charge, as they may be constantly going to be relying on their cherished ones to offer a further layer of safety and protection from the evils of the real worldwide.

Spiritual Values

White Aura power presentations the mild of GOD, so it is the feeling of the divine internal. It pertains to excessive Spiritual power. It connects people with Angelic geographical regions and as a substitute prolonged religious authorities. In maximum of the pix, the halo has been depicted by means of manner of white gowns and mild throughout the top. In case you are capable of take a look at white auric emissions from a person, then it is high quality that there's some spiritual which means that or hyperlink to it. This feature is intrinsically linked to purity, this is why maximum religions use the colour white, in particular symbolically, to thing purity.

Gold auras be part of properly to White Auras, as people with every are generally pure of spirit and is probably related to the spirit global. If someone consists of a white and gold air of mystery, they're taken into consideration to be guided via a higher power, and you'll hook up with this strength at one-of-a-kind instances, like at the same time as you meditate to acquire a diploma of enlightenment.

A individual that consists of a continuously White Aura normally has reached the very great ranges of enlightenment. They embody every spiritual figures and everyday residents, but they will be willing to be beyond tough over earthly troubles and as a substitute purpose better tiers of being. They're often featured with grace of their actions.

CLEANSING YOUR AURA

Now that we are aware about our Aura, we recognize that over a time body we create or acquire dirt or say anomalies in our Aura. So, now can be the time to preserve your attention out of your busy schedules to pay interest and dedicate it to your self, for the restructuring of your Aura, to benefit the advantages defined for us.

Attention and cleansing of Aura may be completed thru severa strategies, including the balancing of your chakra gadget. These unbalanced chakras are revealed in a unmarried's Aura, but it's far hard to find out that a possible imbalance exists; and because of that occasionally, one simply feels out of kinds. At instances they do not apprehend wherein the ones emotions are coming from, which in turn creates a entire unawareness concerning the imbalance. So whether or not or not or not or now not there is an imbalance, it's far a awesome concept to cleanse it often, in reality in case any terrible energies intend to stay indoors.

Remember, there can be no unmarried manner to cleanse your Aura, on the way to try out a few techniques and use the most effective that feels suitable to them. Some of my tips or personal favorites are:

Meditation/Mindfulness

Meditation comes from Latin phrases: meditari (to anticipate, to stay upon, to exercise the thoughts) and mederi (to heal). Some accept as actual with that the word has been derived from the Sanskrit word 'Medha' which shows attention.

Many humans feel doing everyday prayers or worship is a gadget of meditation. But, they want to recognize that meditation is more than that; it's miles honestly now not limited to our each day prayers. It is ready hobby. Anything and everything you do with recognition are considered meditation. Watching your breath is a shape of meditation, and is the most usually taught and simplest to research. Listening to birds, playing the sound of waterfalls or raindrops are few others to name. As prolonged as the ones sports activities are unfastened from any form of distraction to the thoughts, it's miles meditation.

It is a very robust but smooth way that allows the aware thoughts to come upon the silent depths of its non-public nature. If you do not forget and are in search of the advantages of this, it appears more then a way; it will become a Way of existence.

It describes a nation of recognition whilst the thoughts is freed from scattered issues and outstanding preparations. The observer (one who is doing meditation) realizes that every interest of the mind is decreased to as a minimum one. Nowadays, it's miles commonly taken as a form of religious workout in which one sits down with eyes closed and empties the thoughts to gain internal peace, rest, or probably an experience with God. Some human beings point out their act of doing a little aspect is a meditation to them, for instance, my friend makes use of the term "Driving automobile is a meditation to me " or "Gardening is my meditation", as a cease result growing confusion or false impression.

Here we offer you with 5 smooth steps for doing meditation so that you can help you in clearing your Aura.

Step 1 Choose a silent area in which you aren't being disturbed and stay a protracted manner from your digital gadgets, mainly your mobile phones and first-rate gadgets that usually pressure your attention away. Now take a seat in a comfortable and snug function, close to your eyes, and take severa deep breaths that will help you concentrate. Breathing is a completely vital technique as with respiration, we are channelizing the pranas in our body. So whilst you breathe in (it's far to be completed thru nostrils), revel in your chest getting stuffed up and belly bloating up with the Air. When liberating the breath (performed thru the mouth), it need to be launched slowly and your chest getting down and the belly moreover gets inside in the direction of the spine.

Step 2 Feel the energies deep interior; don't forget the electricity interior you is developing with every breath you are taking, till it fills you up out of your ft to the crown of your head. You can enjoy every vein, every blood mobile filled up with this electricity, and charging every mobile of the body. Feel each cell in your frame vibrating with this new electricity they got. Relax your stomach and let any anxiety go together with the waft out with the breath you exhale. You can also strive sending all stress and tension to mother earth. For doing that sense the power targeted to your frame - feel your legs, your decrease body open, and ship all of the anxiety you deliver downwards out of your legs to your toes and further to the ground. Continue doing this for a while till you experience which you are in a place of stillness.

Step-three Bring your attention slowly and consciously to each chakra of your frame from root to crown, and believe the colours in the ones regions getting easy. You will feel the vibration of these chakras getting higher and higher with time, and getting stronger, increasing in duration and beginning.

Step-4 Imagine that the sunbeams radiating out of your coronary coronary heart are stretching from your frame and filling your body with love and slight. Take yourself into the pleasure of this new electricity you are producing and feel like you're floating with this electricity, and brightness is all around you.

Step-5 When you are prepared, permit all of the snap shots dissolve slowly and are to be had lower returned in your popularity. Bring your self once more into your body, respiratory slowly. Feel your palms, your legs, your toes, your palms, and begin feeling that you are right here, to your physical body, related to the ground. When you revel in you're prepared, slowly open your eyes. And now touch your body from head to toe as you are brushing your body together collectively with your fingers.

The higher the vibration of someone, the effective strength they might sense spherical.

Using Aromatherapy

Aromatherapy, the era of the usage of scents and fragrances to assist heal and remove negativity from our our our bodies is in use for loads of years. Using flower fragrances, scents, wild herbs, and woods is the satisfactory and only way for cleansing Aura.

It is a complete technique that makes use of herbal plant extracts to beautify fitness and nicely-being. It is typically referred to as essential oil remedy. This technique makes use of fragrant important oils medicinally to decorate the fitness of the frame, thoughts, and spirit. It facilitates each physical and emotional health and stimulates the thoughts, adjustments moods, and enables religious elevation with the aid of using stimulating the chakras.

Aromatherapy is taken into consideration as each arts and technological information. In the ultra-modern beyond, it has gained an awful lot popularity in the fields of era and remedy. Scents from flower extracts, wild herbs, and woods are the herbal mediums for air of mystery cleaning. A surprising alternate of perfume can energize or relax, can shake emotions, or supply yet again happiness. Focus to your breath and visualize the healing electricity of the perfume is taking over. Within this, I determine on the use of Aromatherapy Based Mist Sprays. I use Emanation AURA CLEANSER and Chakra Balancer Mist Sprays.

These mist sprays are made with a aggregate of different factors and strategies. As inside the making of these sprays Gex Elixir, Holy water from the Ganges, Deep Meditation Energies, Mantra Energies, Color Therapy, and Crystals energies are used, and then those are all home made and organized in small batches with love and affection. My non-public enjoy with these products may be very a success, and people have been very effective and beneficial in clearing awful energy from my subjects. This horrible power can get trapped to your Aura, domestic, or workplace and can were transferred from certainly one of a type human beings with whom we engage. May be from regions we stay/lived or in which we paintings/worked, or journey in/to, from modern-day or vintage feelings that we have now not genuinely released. Lower energies may have an effect on sincerely every body, specifically in the path of times of excessive-strain and transition.

Sometimes we entice, get hold of, and absorb decrease energies from people or in our environment. This electricity can weigh you down and have an impact for your emotion. Releasing it assist you to & the best that you love's experience lighter & happier, balanced, focused, grounded, loving & open. Clearing it from residing & running areas moreover will let you loosen up. Tune in, communicate with others, & create success more effects.

Chapter 8: The Science And Energy Of The Aura

What Science Tells Us about Auras

Einstein and specific physicists have clarified that, at the nuclear level, all matters that exist in nature are electricity, fluctuating and resounding at outstanding frequencies. Some of these active oscillations are widely recognized, along with moderate or sound, radio waves, or X-rays, every reverberating at a particular rhythm.

Human beings and our surrounding auras additionally encompass electricity, with vibrations as particular as fingerprints. And, like anywhere, the strength surges: inner our our our bodies as emotions, or maybe externally, when giving or changing information. Our strength is altered with the aid of way of outside conditions, through emotions and mind, and the alternative is likewise proper. Every act that one initiates is felt as a pulse thru the environment. Energy works like that, and each fluctuation will have an effect on the times of the whole lot that surrounds us: all our deeds, mind, phrases, and beliefs assemble and shape our worldwide – and even our our our bodies.

There had been severa clinical research carried out inside the remaining hundred years, concerning the man or woman of this energy and its capability makes use of.

In the 1930s, Russian researcher Semyon Kirlian implemented a immoderate-frequency electric powered current to a coin, and an photo become produced, displaying a luminous glow across the object, indicating that there is probably a surrounding power area.

Many scientists argue that the Kirlian photo and certainly one of a kind similar photographs are excellent the outcomes of electrical discharge, and no longer a true example of an air of secrecy.

Others thing out that there may be no clinical confirmation to assist the concept that auras have any practical or therapeutic makes use of. Such claims are not supported with the aid of scientific proof and are consequently taken into consideration pseudoscience.

But, presently, in a check published inside the Journal of Conscious and Cognition[1] that unveils why healers see human auras, a set of Spanish researchers from the University of Granada found that lots of folks that claim to peer the auras of numerous men and women are synesthetes: they've greater pass-wiring synaptic links inside the brain than everyday, causing them to make uncommon establishments. They can experience flavors, taste or see sounds, or combine women and men with sun shades. This neuro- and psychologic phenomenon is called synesthesia and is once in a while gift among healers and artists. This capability offers them emotion and pain-analyzing competencies and masses of empathy, despite the fact that the specialists don't don't forget it an extrasensory capability, however as an alternative a beautified and subjective effect of the actual global.

Despite the controversies, exceptional research considered that a promising place of research is the use of magnetic resonance imaging (MRI) and thermal imaging to visualise the distribution and adjustments inside the frame's energy vicinity. These strategies attempt to find out unique areas of the air of mystery which may be related to incredible components of physical and highbrow health.

The studies moreover maintains at the therapeutic functionality of some strategies which use frame power, like Reiki, meditation, and considered one of a kind mindfulness practices in improving fitness.

Of course, more scientific efforts are needed to apprehend the character of the aura and its capacity uses. However, present day technology and new proof recommend that the electricity area surrounding the body is a real and probably useful phenomenon that merits similarly studies.

Energy Centers and the Aura

Energy facilities are energy facilities that generate electricity for the specific regions of the body. Also referred to as chakras, which in Sanskrit translates to "wheel" or "disk," they may be the wheels of energy at a few level within the frame, the access factors for existence power. Their shape is like plant life made from slight. They correspond to numerous organs and glands of the frame primarily based on their positions.

Ancient artifacts mean that chakras are believed to be spheroid electricity spirals in the frame, rotating and soaking up healthful strength from outside, whilst discharging horrible electricity from the indoors. The chakras are described as electricity packing containers or electricity stations responsible for shelling out existence pressure at some diploma inside the body. Depending at the strength we collect and comprise, we can be greater healthful, happier, and well internal, and assignment appropriate waves externally.

A sturdy chakra is whirling rapid, and not using a blockages to forestall the circulate of power that we want to stay. But chakras are not constantly in particular situation, and they're all of the time shifting and enhancing. Their state is predicated upon on many instances, together with their manner of existence, idea system, emotional research, and kismet. As one actions through lifestyles sports, the chakras are assimilating those impacts.

The human frame has seven vital chakras, aligned from the pinnacle of the top to the lowest of the vertebral column, seven whirling electricity stations with their very own one among a kind attributes, much like the colors of the spectrum: Violet, Indigo, Blue, Green, Yellow, Orange, and Red.

Let's take a look at the electricity facilities within the human frame:

ROOT CHAKRA

Located genuinely under the perineum, it's far like a root of a tree, and, if it's robust, the person can be robust and wholesome.

Physical important locus: the lowest of the spinal column.

Allied with balance, safety, protection, survival, foundation, inherited ideals, popularity of affinity to a hard and fast and to a location, adrenal glands – the "combat or flight" reaction to conditions, the choice to stay, the skeletal and muscular structures, the manufacturing of blood, and the number one layer or the air of mystery.

When balanced, we experience included and loved in the international, we are grounded, and our frame gets an terrific waft of power.

When imbalanced, we experience annoying, disconnected, and compelled. We revel in a lack of grounding and sleep deprivation.

Weaknesses: sciatica, similarly to ingesting and immune issues.

Beneficial crystals: tourmaline, garnet, hematite, obsidian, jasper.

SACRAL CHAKRA

Located at the pinnacle of the sacrum, beneath the navel.

Physical primary locus: decrease stomach proper beneath the navel.

Allied with feelings, relationships, growing concord or disharmony, sensuality, sexuality, strength, creativity, the astral or emotional body, the inner baby, the reproductive glands, the functionality to experience delight, being open to exchange, new mind and reviews, and the second layer of the charisma.

When balanced, we are able to articulate our emotions and ardour in a healthy way, and the mild of the soul is truly pondered.

When imbalanced, we endure emotional capriciousness or sexual flaws, we experience inflexible and may't cope with trade.

Weaknesses: sexual organ afflictions, guilt, sexual repression, shame, urinary problems, emotions, relationships, and cash problems.

Beneficial crystals: amber, calcite, carnelian, citrine, moonstone.

SOLAR PLEXUS CHAKRA

Located inside the location of the diaphragm, the various ribs and in the again.

Physical fundamental locus: stomach, above the navel, and below the sternum.

Allied with movement, non-public energy, will, courage, self notion, power of will, arrogance, aim, intestine emotions/don't forget, power, ego, liver, pancreas, spleen, diaphragm, belly, the great of blood, appendix, intestines, coronary heart, lungs, the heating and cooling tool of the body, the seat of stress, and the third layer of the air of thriller.

When balanced, we sense confident and on top of things of our destinies, the ego is aligned with the Higher Self.

When imbalanced, we enjoy powerless, lack self-appreciate and self assurance, adopt a "me in competition to the others" mentality, grievance, judgments, separation, fear exclusion, and problem attaining conclusions.

Weaknesses: abuse, acid reflux disorder, adrenal issues, tension, horrible emotions within the pit of the belly, exhaustion, fatigue, want to dominate, gall bladder problems, irritable bowels.

Beneficial crystals: amber, citrine, jasper, tiger's eye.

HEART CHAKRA

Located on the center of the chest.

Physical essential locus: lungs and coronary coronary heart, arms, fingers.

Allied with presenting and receiving, compassion, (self-)forgiveness, (self-)love, empathy, compassion, releasing past hurts, the thymus gland, and the circulatory tool, which regulates the immune function, and the fourth layer of the air of mystery.

When balanced, we are capable of bestow and get preserve of affection, and we apprehend that what's right for one is proper for all.

When imbalanced, we meet adversities in our relationships, we sense disconnected from others, and feel an absence of love.

Weaknesses: allergic reactions, congestion or coronary heart failure, grief, guilt, coronary heart attack, heartbreak, pneumonia, tuberculosis, resentments, loss of potential to sympathize and empathize.

The 1/three and fourth chakras are right now associated: while the zero.33 is over-energized, it depletes the fourth.

Beneficial crystals: malachite, quartz, tourmaline.

THROAT CHAKRA

Located on the middle of the neck.

Physical fundamental locus: mouth, thyroid, throat.

Allied with preference, the functionality to give or exchange information openly and sincerely, self-expression, and creativity, the thyroid gland, which runs the metabolism, the parathyroid glands and the lymphatic device, and the 5th layer of the charisma.

When balanced, we're capable of communicate and speak the fact, we're related to our soul and capable of create or take place.

When imbalanced, we aren't clean about what to do or a manner to pass ahead, communicate with difficulty, we may be dishonest, over-active or under-lively, enjoy like we're not being understood, and feature trouble finding the proper terms.

Weaknesses: addictions, being essential and judgmental, loss of voice, bronchial allergies, sore throat, swollen glands, goiter, thyroid issues, sterility.

The fifth and second chakras are without delay related; over-hobby inside the sacral chakra depletes the throat chakra, dropping communique capabilities, our course to knowledge, or the connection with the soul.

Beneficial crystals: agate, aquamarine, calcite, turquoise.

THIRD EYE CHAKRA

Located many of the eyes.

Physical number one locus: the middle of the forehead, cerebellum, pineal gland, ears, and eyes.

Allied with discerning the reality, intuition, open-mindedness, capability to assume abstractly and to look the big photograph, creativeness, foresight, facts, clairvoyance, and information the underlying styles in our lives. It controls and energizes the pituitary gland, which runs the endocrine glands and the brain, the respiration device, eyes and nostril, the recapitulation of all of the strength from the lower chakras, and the sixth layer of the air of mystery.

When balanced, we can have confidence in our intuition and suppose at the start. Like having a 3rd eye, this chakra opens our recognition to the better plane.

When imbalanced, we've got got problems with ingenuity, centering, or desire-making, we are too much in our heads, and we lack purpose.

Weaknesses: blindness, thoughts tumors, deafness, despair, dizziness, complications, odd sleep, mastering disabilities, migraines, paranoia, seizures, strokes, diabetes.

Beneficial crystals: amethyst, fluorite, lapis lazuli, sodalite.

CROWN CHAKRA

Located above the pinnacle.

Physical principal locus: the pinnacle of the pinnacle and the skull, the pituitary gland.

Allied with familiar love, non secular connection to the universe, spirituality, inner steerage, the pouring of divine energy into our machine, reference to the regular reputation and the divine, the understanding that all things are related, controlling and energizing the brain, and the complete frame, and the seventh layer of the air of mystery.

When balanced, we feel wholeness with the world and function a deep popularity of our location in it.

When imbalanced, we enjoy detached from the world or from our non secular selves, we lack cause, and might't locate significance in existence.

Weaknesses: alienation, melancholy, detachment, disconnection, exhaustion, loss of compassion, disturbing device imbalances, and anxiety resulting from sound and moderate.

Beneficial crystals: amethyst, quartz, selenite, topaz.

Decoding the Colors of Your Aura

"Aura" refers to the religious strain of someone. An charisma of a extensive variety will enfold being involved human beings and enlightened spirits. Their energy area may be sensed from a distance.

But sensing an air of mystery is an paintings. As with studying any functionality, you need to exercising. Some trust this have turn out to be natural within the vintage days, however, over the centuries the exercise declined and faded, like many different abilties.

Auras are all unique. As a end result, at the same time as analyzing them we will see all forms of sunglasses, in hundreds of sun sun sunglasses.

The sun shades have which means; they inform us critical matters approximately ourselves. Their places are in direct relation to the chakras, at the same time as their volume, sun sunglasses, and vibration are with regards to the hobby of the unique chakra.

Are there a few sunglasses that are more regular than others? Those who examine auras might provide an reason of that it's far predicated upon on the individual that is the venture of the reading. All hues are taken into consideration wholesome, as long as they'll be ours. A lot of depression comes from bearing air of thriller sunglasses that are not our non-public, however which we revel in forced to position on with the intention to live on.

In auras, the density of colors is the maximum critical thing to have a look at. Each color has a particular rhythm. Red is the minimal, and violet has the tremendous drift.

Aura hues cannot be counterfeit, just so they assist us examine people for what they may be. The sun shades of 1's air of thriller also can assist find out illnesses, health deficiencies, and intellectual confusion.

We've mentioned the seven important colorations regarding the seven chakras of the human frame. There are also sun shades of those hues. Therefore, reading someone's air of mystery intensive can take the time to understand. The hardest detail approximately auras isn't seeing them but analyzing to have a study them. It can be difficult to analyze someone's air of thriller at the beginning due to the fantastic levels of the energy location.

Also, the world of electricity surrounding our bodily frame is stricken by our mood and emotional usa (and the states of others), and specific sunglasses are associated with unique inclinations and emotions all of the time.

An charisma is a combination of colors, with one or being more dominant than others. Also, the charisma can shift and trade relying on one's kingdom of mind, with physical and emotional trauma or illnesses, and as you undergo life and change as a person. Humans are lively and complicated, so we are able to recognize that our auras are simply as complicated and complex as we're.

Aura shades can also seem clean and real or muddied or faded. Both the situation of the colour and the colour itself may advocate amazing components of a person's real individual.

Each colour is associated with first rate strengths and developments. Before figuring out the colors, it's crucial to increase a deeper know-how of auras, belief to be composed of 7 unique auric subtle our our our bodies, or layers of electricity, attaining out past the physical body, every so often as a long manner as three ft or more. The seven power vicinity tiers wrap the human body in a huge oval-fashioned energy trouble.

The Etheric Body is associated with the Root Chakra and is involved with ache and pleasure and the automatic skills of the frame. Extending one to 2 inches out from the bodily frame, it's like webs and small lines of sparkling moderate which may be constantly flowing.

The Emotional Body is related to the Sacral Chakra and is concerned with emotions. Extending one to 3 inches out from the bodily frame, it has no exact colour or shape however is constantly moving.

The Mental Body is associated with the Solar Plexus Chakra and is worried with the intellect and the left mind. Extending 3 to 8 inches out from the bodily body, it is structured with the mind and colored thru the emotion involved.

The Astral Body is related to the Heart Chakra and is concerned with love. Extending 12 inches out from the bodily body, getting towards the astral international and spirits, it consists of pink.

The Etheric Body is related to the Throat Chakra and is worried with divine will and conversation. Extending 12–25 inches out from the individual, it's miles considered the blueprint of the physical frame, and if some other auric body is damaged, the etheric body heals it.

The Celestial Body is associated with the Third Eye Chakra and is worried with celestial love. Extending 24–30 inches out from the bodily body, it may be reached with meditation to heal and speak with our spirit.

The Causal Body is associated with the Crown Chakra and is involved with the higher self, extending 24–36 inches out from the physical frame and shimmering gold and silver.

Remember, no auras are alike. They variety in shade intensity, distribution, and brilliant.

Aura colorings may also display your person and metaphysical development if they're accurately interpreted. Knowing the way to study and determine your air of thriller is every an know-how and an art work. This can be a lifelong studying manner, and this ebook is your first step on the journey.

The energy fields consist of a large number of colors, but one is dominant — and that colour displays the maximum extraordinary tendencies of the being. Anytime a person's air of thriller appears dirty, dark, and cloudy, it's due to the fact terrible energy of some kind is suppressing their actual nature. Maybe the character has tension that stops them from being themselves, or they're concealing some factor. And, no matter the reality that maximum humans's air of mystery is dominated thru using one shade, a few have a aggregate of colours — a mixture of character developments, or even a rainbow — indicating individuals who are stressed, who're going via a big exchange, or who are enlightened.

How Life Experiences Shape Your Aura

Auras do surely alternate and evolve.

There is a major life purpose colour, indicating who an individual is. However, this shade can fade or lose its specific tone, depending on what the character does in their existence. A physical healthy and glad person will possibly have a wonderful, clear, and great charisma.

A man or woman's issues furthermore make a distinction. Artists and passionate people have a tendency to have extra pink, orange, yellow, and crimson. But in the event that they decide to shift their life path and pick out to become mentors or teachers, their power location will probably come to be extra blue and inexperienced.

People with top behavior are extra active, immoderate brilliant, and wholesome and their air of thriller glows. All which you think, trust, say, do, eat, and breathe impacts the energy concern that surrounds your bodily body. Throughout the day, we accomplish, enjoy, and understand numerous topics. Our strength fields will endorse this as properly. Positive emotions will in reality have an impact at the air of mystery, whilst strain and stress may have an effect on it negatively. The situation of the body, emotions, attitudes, thoughts, and contamination affect the electricity scenario, as does religious improvement.

So, existence memories will have a huge impact in your charisma, shaping its color, form, and wellknown strength. It is concept to be a contemplated image of your physical, emotional, and non secular kingdom, and might trade and evolve through the years as you go through precise reminiscences and levels.

Traumatic stories along aspect injuries, ailments, or abuse can depart imprints to your electricity discipline. They display up as dark spots, blockages, or unique irregularities, and may require strength artwork or other healing modalities to cope with.

On the opportunity hand, powerful stories consisting of affection, pleasure, and creativity can also depart imprints of brighter and extra colorful hues. When you feel satisfied, fulfilled, and linked on your authentic purpose, your air of mystery may additionally additionally seem large and brighter.

Ultimately, your air of thriller is a dynamic and ever-evolving meditated photo of your inner and outer worldwide, and its hues and form can give you precious insights into your bodily, emotional, and religious country.

Chapter 9: Reading Auras

The Art of Aura Reading

Since the charisma is found great thru clairvoyance or psychic vision, the interpretation is subjective, relying on the pleasant facts of the reader.

Here are a few vital issues on the identical time as decoding the air of mystery:

the severa regions reflecting the astral, etheric, intellectual, or non secular our our bodies

frame levels similar to the position of the chakras

which colorations appear, and the way easy and intense they're

the presence of patterns or distortions: agitation, arcs, balance, blockages, bulges, clusters, depressions, fissures, fluctuations, holes, elements of darkness or moderate, streaks, streams, symmetry, or tentacles geometric figures

the general shape

the observer's emotions and psychic beliefs.

The air of secrecy reader want first of all some essential troubles of these elements, and next have a take a look at the complexity of the entire air of mystery.

An charisma reader sees styles and feels electricity. Seeing the air of secrecy is one step, however the key's to organize the information and have a look at and interpret observations. By mastering to read auras and facts their shades and meanings, you may regulate your instinct. Through studying auras, you could pick out out why a few people offer you with lousy vibes and why you revel in exquisite round others.

Being able to see auras isn't as out of attain as it would seem. However, it consists of extremely good self-discovery at the start: you should discover ways to see them with the beneficial aid of first studying your very non-public aura. Try this in a room with white walls, and watch your body in a replicate. Look above the pinnacle of your head. Relax your eyes, and stand there for seven mins on the identical time as you empty your thoughts. Soon, you'll see waves of colors. They is probably best in the outer edge of your imaginative and prescient, however don't try to pursue them – allow them to glide as they may. You will start to see your energy area enfolding your frame.

Once you understand a manner to try this, try to see your pals' auras. Eventually, you could boom your capacity as a way to observe the auras of whole strangers.

Before lengthy, it will evolve right into a dependancy!

Remember that the color of your air of thriller will shift and exchange because of the truth the power is flowing. But humans don't make huge modifications or adjust their way of life often, so drastic adjustments are unusual.

When your air of thriller appears to come to be cloudy or dirty, it need to be a take into account of interest – however don't panic. With reflected picture, rest, and self-love, your aura can be wiped easy and more potent over again.

Aura readings are useful for staying focused and ensuring that you're feeling calm and accumulated. If some issue is off, there may be a contradictory strength you're radiating which you aren't even aware of. Or perhaps you're permitting some foreign places energies to steer you extra than you understand.

You can have your air of mystery photographed the usage of a special digital digicam referred to as the AuraCam 6000. It come to be created within the 1970s – but the exercise of air of mystery snap shots come to be initiated within the Nineteen

Thirties, via the Russian electric powered engineer, Semyon Kirlian.

If you depend high-quality on the pix approach, you'll possibly get a as a substitute superficial analyzing, in comparison with what you may acquire if you go to an air of mystery reader in character. A picture will no longer display any electricity or movement to your air of thriller; as with any image, it captures the dominion of your charisma at one immediately in time.

Sometimes the charisma may also additionally moreover appear very huge, irrespective of the truth that duration differs from one individual to every other and may exchange. Whenever we meet with excellent humans, our energy fields 'amalgamate, and – whether or now not or no longer we are privy to it – we understand warning symptoms from distinct human beings's auras all the time.

Although we won't recognize it, every body use our auras as detection machine. Maybe in the beyond, you've felt like someone modified into looking you, or perhaps you've got got felt drawn to a specific person, and also you weren't fine why. Have you ever felt distressed even as fame in a specific vicinity, no matter the fact that you'd never been there earlier than? These topics take area while your energy area is reacting to each reciprocal or communicate energies. You may additionally moreover have called this "instinct," or a "intestine feeling."

You don't want specific gadget to hit upon power fields, you can use dowsing rods or pendulums, and that similarly they may be perceived with the arms – as we see dowsing rods, which react to the holder's strength problem.

The satisfactory motive to discover ways to take a look at auras is to help you study your self and others, so you can live existence extra truly.

It can also make an effort and a few tries to look your air of thriller, however as fast as you've got were given perceived your strength difficulty, we're capable of input the following degree. Now, we learn to discern the colours and their meanings.

A Colorful Guide to Common Aura Meanings

The air of secrecy, or the energy problem that surrounds the human body, is often described in phrases of shade. Each coloration indicates a special problem of an man or woman's physical, emotional, and spiritual properly-being. Your air of thriller may be a single shade or a mixture. Multiple sun shades really imply which you're experiencing more than one emotion on the identical time.

Red

RED is the bottom frequency colour at the spectrum, related to the earth and the bodily aircraft.

Focus: base of the backbone and the primal ROOT CHAKRA, related to foundational elements, easy goals, and reference to the physical body and the tangible global.

RED aura phrases: adrenaline, agitation, anger, blood, air of mystery, cherries, determination, strain, exhaustion, issues with the circulatory and breathing device, management, excitement, outbursts of anger (seeing red), red roses, obligation, sensuality, sexual desires, sexual electricity, energy, robust emotions, trauma, electricity.

RED air of thriller trends: dramatic, athlete, famous via many, adventurous, aggressive, ambitious, courageous, competitive, confident, courageous, direct and to-the-factor, dynamic, active, enthusiastic, fearless, fiery, annoyed, purpose-oriented, hyper-stimulated, impulsive, individualistic, unstable, challenger, overworked, passionate, pressured, sturdy, realistic, violent, and now not the usage of a hidden time desk.

RED aura people want to every act by myself or be in charge of others and shine as leaders, in any other case, they turn out to be overbearing. They located pretty a few try into how they look. Easily bored, they get bored halfway through the obligations they begin. They confuse lust for romance in relationships, inflicting warfare and damage, being horrible and jealous at the same time as topics don't move their way. It's difficult to win at the same time as you move them. They are effective with a zest for existence, and they typically generally tend to overindulge in easy pleasures. They come off as wholesome because of the reality they workout and characteristic toned our our bodies. Grounded in their dreams, they need wealth, and feature a laugh spending cash and experiencing many adventures. Passion and restlessness maintain them pushed and that they seem unafraid of risks or lack of existence. They speedy placed their mind into movement and do not test training manuals. They rate subjects they may touch, see, pay attention, and flavor. They love exploring fantastic locations and that they have got a formidable method to existence. Their enjoy of adventure isn't limited to excursion, however additionally meals and intercourse. They cost physical connections, intimacy, cash, and adventure. Their lust for lifestyles can be channeled for the wrong motives and lead them astray.

Orange

ORANGE indicates self assurance, creativity, what makes you precise, and a satisfied exchange of power, love, cash, property, time, or artwork.

Focus: genital or SACRAL CHAKRA, the power center for creativity and sexual power, of trade and relationships, of valuing friendships and social interplay.

ORANGE aura terms: creativity, egotism, enthusiasm, frustration, fun, appropriate fitness, reproductive machine or digestion problems, delight, openness, sensuality, and power.

ORANGE charisma trends: affectionate, fascinating, infant-like, competitive, emotional, unfastened-energetic, beneficiant, gregarious, sincere, impatient, independent, type, constructive, human beings-pleaser, persuasive, sociable, spontaneous, diffused, and volatile.

ORANGE charisma human beings rush into tasks or relationships rapid without questioning them through, appearing first and handling the effects later. Optimistic, angered, impatient, chance-taking, and obsessive, pursuing new hobbies and pursuits with willpower, dwelling every day find it impossible to resist's their final, we will be part of them on their journey in the fast lane or be exceeded thru way of. Quick to forgive and without keeping grudges, they'll be properly and charismatic leaders. They do properly in plenty of workplaces however being brave, they pick out better-risk jobs, like firefighting and navy. Or, being extroverts, they pursue careers with more social interplay, like politics and earnings. With appropriate health and lots of energy, constantly trying a present day exercising venture, they may be predisposed to be in a incredible mood, so that they just get along element others and make buddies without problems. They deliver strength to their groups due to being relatable and sociable, studying instructions from experience, the tough way, in area of from precept. Daredevils who are looking for for out the thrill and amusing in any scenario, don't sit down however as they want to experience all the global has to offer and apprehend their authentic nature and stay creatively, craving newness and sensation, which may additionally furthermore reason dependancy or hassle committing in relationships. Perceptive and dynamic, their relationships increase fast. They personal a disarming first-rate that places others relaxed; they love being within the commercial enterprise agency of numerous people, are happy with their circle of relatives, friends, and surroundings, and are outstanding present givers because of the fact they understand the mind and feelings of others.

Yellow

YELLOW is awakening, inspirational and colourful, sunny and vibrant, completely satisfied, awesome, and powerful.

Focus: the SOLAR PLEXUS CHAKRA, related to intellect, amusing, optimism and notion, self-esteem and personal strength, identity, and self assurance.

YELLOW aura terms: summary questioning, balance, brightness, cheerfulness, clarity, communication, dependability, digestive tool troubles, egoism, happiness, hunger for greatness, internal happiness, mind, lack of power, mechanical abilties, highbrow electricity, overconfidence, perfectionism, self-complaint, conceitedness, social competence, spiritual awakening, sun, sunflowers, superior eye-hand coordination, verbal skills, and information.

YELLOW air of thriller tendencies: analytical, appealing, bossy, charismatic, confident, innovative, empowered, free, complete of existence, smart, joyous, magnetic, wonderful, playful, problem-fixing, prolific author, radiant, smart, active, strong personality, sunny, talkative, heat, and witty.

YELLOW air of mystery humans inspire others to attain greatness. They are born leaders with a lot energy and the capability to encourage, they encourage and aid others through manner of manner of being themselves and radiating just like the solar.

Full of generosity and inner joy, they prefer to have a laugh and don't take existence too notably, attracting others within the direction of them, and preserving positions of strength, being managers, politicians, administrators, or dad and mom.

Always in the avant-garde, they suppose unconventionally and aren't afraid to test. They can examine complicated standards, strolling in teaching and studies careers, as inventors, scientists, or professors, as they will be moreover fantastic communicators, assured each in a unmarried-on-one situations further to inside the front of a crowd.

Tending to overwork themselves and valuing careers above relationships, they don't have any trouble being on their non-public, even maintaining apart themselves at the equal time as compelled. With immoderate belief and being very critical of themselves and others, they have got a look at and observe human beings and feature just a few however fine friendships, because of the truth they provide a deep love. They supply fun into day by day existence and make it higher for others. They also realise while to get to paintings, but don't enjoy meaningless duties; they need to make contributions to something massive than themselves. They partner with human beings like themselves: modern and smart.

Green

GREEN is the color of plants, outside, connection to nature, alternate, and boom.

Focus: the HEART CHAKRA, associated with private increase and self-actualization, healing energy, love, affinity with nature, international situations challenge, and compassion.

GREEN air of thriller phrases: stability, envy (green with envy), adversity, catastrophe, growth, coronary coronary heart or immune machine troubles, contamination, inner war, jealousy, overcoming boundaries, realistic worldview, resistance to exchange, subjects of the heart, open coronary coronary heart, self-love, and love for others.

GREEN air of thriller dispositions: calm, being concerned, compassionate, revolutionary, decided, down-to-earth, empathetic, focused, forgiving, healer, impatient, nurturing, open, perfectionist, for my part unfulfilled, self-assertive, serene, now not positive, with immoderate beliefs and aspirations.

Influenced by using the usage of way in their environment, GREEN aura human beings love tune, now not being tied down, and nature, getting out, going tenting, or walking within the park. They have type hearts, and love animals, plants, pals, family, and all life. They deliver equal interest to their own desires and to the human beings they love, radiating unconditional love and a life pressure strength that is sensed via all beings. Their presence is non violent and restful. They may be nurses, healers, instructors, mother and father, and environmentalists; they display duty and issuer to others, bridging the religious and bodily worlds. They are healers with out even understanding it, recovery the soul with their phrases, and are often writers. They preserve stability by using using adapting to exchange, staying far from unrealistic mind, and doing well with buddies and companions who also are relaxed. Influenced by means of the use of way of various human beings, they may normally have a tendency to sense like a sufferer and reflect onconsideration on remarks from others as grievance, this is why boundaries are essential for them. They act because of the fact the referee in private relationships, stuck in others' dramas and interpersonal conflicts till they get worn out with the resource of manner in their efforts to mediate. Their creativity manifests in new and sensible strategies, crafting, gardening, cooking, and redecorating the house. Wiser than maximum, they're the "vintage souls." Green air of thriller people are a hit in industrial enterprise agency (and any pastime) due to the reality they're planners who don't love to do rash subjects, however, they will change their desires frequently. They are well-known and revered with the useful resource of coworkers, partners, and friends.

Blue

BLUE is associated with the verbal exchange.

Focus: THROAT CHAKRA, controlling expression, and talking one's truth.

BLUE charisma phrases: balance, conversation, compassion, despondency, emotional manipulate, empathy, feeling blue, flexibility, honesty, loss of self perception, meditation, optimism, peace, pessimism, self-expression, self-perception, serenity, pressure, throat or thyroid problems, and quietness.

BLUE air of thriller dispositions: alert, calm, disturbing, assured, creative, expressive, intuitive, touchy, religious, suicidal, and witty.

BLUE charisma people take existence more appreciably. They place fee on their own family and pals and protect those they care approximately. Expressive and succesful to mention what they have got of their minds, can with out problem supply mind, mind, perspectives, and thoughts to pals and strangers alike; they are public audio system, politicians, singers, philosophers, poets, and writers.

They have intelligence and notion and be given as authentic with their emotions to determine what's suitable with out requiring outdoor facts. Integrity and accuracy in communique are critical to them. They need to extract and percentage information. They task peaceful and exquisite electricity.

With effective minds, but a chunk inside the clouds, they perform greater within the intellectual geographical areas and want to floor themselves. But further they'll be insightful, proudly proudly owning instinct, highbrow readability, and being inwardly centered.

Great listeners, who usually appear to have the fantastic recommendation. Creative and artistic in a few manner, they live their lives in a unique manner than maximum.

Workaholics take on an excessive amount of proper now. Scared by way of way of way of their very very personal sensitivity and vulnerability, it's tough to get to understand them.

Indigo

INDIGO represents deep instinct.

Focus: BROW CHAKRA, associated with spiritual popularity, inner understanding, connection to the better self, experience of cause, and challenge.

INDIGO aura phrases: dreaming, empathy, pineal gland problems, self-doubt, and uncertainty.

INDIGO aura tendencies: communicator, connector, modern, disconnected, introverted, intuitive, seeker, touchy, religious, and visionary.

INDIGO air of thriller humans have a strong instinct and that they're curious, constantly learning and attempting to find the truth. In music with their higher self, they might experience distinct human beings's energies, seeing beyond deceit and lies. They can experience matters in advance than they take area, or recognize what someone will say in advance than they communicate.

They stay in the present and go together with the go with the float, basing their alternatives at the depth in their feelings.

They assist others to understand the grace and the immensity of nature and its secrets and techniques and techniques and strategies, soaking up the feelings, emotions, thoughts, and traumas of others.

They personal advanced verbal abilities and command appreciate, getting pretty a few hobby because of their instinct, sensitivity, and first rate highbrow depth.

Being in a position to connect to others effects leads humans to understand and admire the splendor of the sector. They should art work in which their empathy can do the notable. With their summary pursuits, they may be theoreticians, philosophers, ministers, and psychics. Wealth consists of them and that they settle into snug careers which permit them to pursue non-public pastimes.

Violet

VIOLET is associated with divine strength, and consequently the farthest some distance from earth.

Focus: CROWN CHAKRA, linked to our fantasies and higher focus, seeing the big photograph, and guiding others to their maximum capacity.

VIOLET air of mystery terms: compassion, connection to the divine, preference to assist others, need to get higher or rest, pineal gland problems, sensitivity, deep spirituality, and immoderate-tempo vibration.

VIOLET air of mystery developments: imaginative, charismatic, dynamic, intuitive, liberal, open-minded, effective persona, modern, spiritual, and sensible.

VIOLET Aura humans are religious leaders or healers with magical and uncommon power, an open 1/three eye, and psychic abilties. They command and encourage others, guiding them right into a modern-day era of prosperity, pleasure, and contentment. They have a very robust desire to carry out some issue essential in their existence. They are visionaries with notable ideals and ambition. Possessing both instinct and records, they may maintain close all of the components of a situation. Effortlessly assessing the vibrations of various people, they desire very an entire lot to connect, inspire, and encourage sharing with others, however they're often unreadable themselves. They may have an off-placing air of superiority and be worried in metaphysical interests. They stay with their head in the clouds, daydreaming and fantasizing. They have robust intestine feelings and their empathy and know-how are valued. In near contact with the cosmos and invisible types of power, questioning lots, and manifesting their predictions into the environment, similarly they display excessive originality, resourceful thoughts, modern-day thoughts, and a thoughts that is open to the universe. However, they every so often battle to speak and won't understand a manner to answer to humans once they acquire unconscious signs. They may additionally exhaust themselves through providing too much to their career or relationships, and that they've problem establishing limitations.

In harmony with the emotions and attitudes of others, they have a profound dating with the herbal environment and animals. Sensitive and mysterious with countless ability for character and religious improvement, their passion for obtaining facts and exploring makes them attractive and knowledgeable. They can see greater than the cloth global.

Other Colors

A PINK air of secrecy is rare. It is related to affection, compassion, love, sweetness, teens, durability, rejuvenation, sensitivity, idealism, abilties, tenderness, warm temperature, peace, and harmony. These humans are romantic, gentle, kind, being involved, empathetic, humanitarian, and nurturing. They use international own family members to give up fights in advance than they even begin, and have a tendency to be happy and in concord with everyone. People need to be around them and their calming and sort power, their open and receptive hearts. They have hundreds love to present however need to installation some barriers. They inspire, comfort, and uplift others of their challenges, recovery them with a glance, a grin, a type word, or really by way of using being gift. They remind us to be gentle with every other and all of earth's creatures. They stay a balanced life between the fabric international and the spiritual international.

A MAGENTA air of thriller is an indication of originality. Independent, revolutionary, unique, progressive, and funny, they've plenty electricity, simply so they don't observe tendencies – they cause them to.

Peer stress doesn't have an effect on them. Considered bizarre and whimsical, they're furthermore stylish because they are uncommon. They experience the arena of their very private manner, surprising special people and shaking up their everyday existence. Optimistic and searching at lifestyles with humor, they'll be strong-willed and wise but not often understood.

People with a BROWN air of secrecy are logical, sensible, robust, dependable, organized, unbiased, and rooted in truth – however additionally greedy and self-absorbed. They constantly have a strict rate range and a detailed prolonged-term career plan, and difficult paintings and method gets them there. With strong pursuits within the out of doors, the Earth, and natural assets, they love operating with their palms and are inquisitive about archaeology, production, ecology, gardening, geology, trekking, looking, snowboarding, and mountain climbing.

A BLACK air of thriller is a sign of anger, despair, emptiness, worry, grief, sick health, lack of purpose, and negativity. These people are feeling out of vicinity or uncertain, exhausted, or fatigued. They need time to liven up, stability, heal, forgive, and allow circulate of their suffering.

GRAY is the shadow of adversity, fitness problems, contamination, or even demise.

WHITE is uncommon. It technique purity, truth, enlightenment, peace, concord, and stability – a connection to a few aspect massive, to the divine, not unusual electricity, and oneness. These humans are religious leaders or healers, angelic or prophetic, perfectionists, and healthy, with a short mind and plenty energy. They don't care lots for fabric possessions or earthly wishes. They are transcending the constraints of the physical realm. Free from personal issues, worldly subjects, or ambition, they may be incredible, uplifting, and non-judgmental, characterized by way of inner illumination and searching for cosmic answers.

While hardly ever seen, SILVER in an air of secrecy method every non secular and material abundance in a life whole of mystery and magic. More dreamers than doers, they may be intuitive and visionary, but impractical.

People with GOLD in their air of mystery are related to the divine energy supply of the universe. They have committed their lifestyles to spirituality and boom. You enjoy at domestic and respected spherical them. They are charismatic and able to deal with big-scale tasks, but they reap their successes later in existence.

The which means of air of secrecy colors is subjective and may vary relying on the man or woman and the cultural context wherein they're interpreted. Also, the interpretation of air of thriller shades can also additionally moreover exchange over time as an character's studies and perceptions evolve, so it's essential to have an open thoughts.

Whether you're a pro practitioner of air of secrecy interpretation or are clearly beginning to find out this charming issue, this colourful guide to common charisma meanings offers an area to begin for know-how the air of thriller and an individual's bodily, emotional, and spiritual properly-being.

Analyzing Aura Patterns

The varieties of energy that surround the human frame may be analyzed to gain perception into someone's bodily, emotional, and non secular properly-being. This effects in a deeper know-how of the individual and gives possibilities for guidance.

Here are the steps:

Before you start studying others, it's far essential to first recognize your very non-public air of secrecy and energy patterns. You can do that thru meditating and becoming privy to your strength and how it feels.

Become acquainted with the super air of mystery patterns, each associated with incredible elements of bodily, emotional, and non secular health. It's vital to apprehend what they imply to analyze the charisma as it have to be.

Open your thoughts and visualize the aura and its one-of-a-kind strength patterns, through meditation, guided visualization wearing activities, or via the usage of aura snap shots.

Pay attention to physical sensations on your body: tingling, warm temperature, or strain in positive regions can imply outstanding components of the air of thriller.

Interpret the patterns. Consider the man or woman's physical, emotional, and non secular nation, and each different applicable factors, to decide what the air of mystery's styles might be telling you approximately their fitness and nicely-being.

Based to your assessment of the air of thriller, you may provide guidance and guidelines, collectively with meditation or electricity recovery, to help balance and enhance their air of secrecy.

Each air of mystery reader sees auras in a totally precise way, with colours and sun sun shades, but additionally shapes and textures. These are the manifestations of energy, reflecting your feature on the time they will be visible, changing, developing, disappearing, and reforming, even as your predominant air of thriller colour and trends stay solid at some point of your existence.

The shapes can show additives of the strength this is coming in and leaving with the feelings of existence: anxiety, depression, pride, disappointment, and marvel – each drawing a particular shape of power and having its personal physical feeling.

Bands: persuasion, leadership, religion. This energy may be applied without a doubt or adversely, based totally on colour: notable to nearly apparent is immoderate first-class; darkish and opaque propose that it'll likely be used with prejudice.

Stars and sparks can stand up anywhere in the energy task, suggesting the want for approval. Based on electricity and area, crimson sparks at the forestall of the vertebral column are an illustration that the character doesn't feel as famous as everyday and is worrying; yellow technique lack of private appreciation regarding modern-day capabilities or sexual dreams; white, silver, and gold recommend the intervention of powerful forces – a spiritual, luminous presence – an angel, or each other advanced guiding force. The people know that a few factor is coming; they just don't understand what, but they experience endowed with some of well electricity.

Dark factors are the reverse of stars, signifying an assault on the air of thriller that wants to be repelled or cleansed: emotional blocks, trauma, infection, damage, loss of electricity, and damaging connections with folks who want to be cleared away from your life.

Voids are inactive areas with very little electricity – empty, lifeless patches revealing discouragement, hopelessness, and detachment. They may be analyzed steady with the area wherein they are found. They want to be eliminated. Untreated, they result in infection.

Whirlpools advise broken relationships, unresolved conflicts, fear, lack of self guarantee, anxiety, and pain within the vicinity wherein they will be visible.

Symmetries are signs and symptoms of a harmonious thoughts, body, and spirit, displaying that someone is able to accommodate modifications which can be occurring and is viewing them as learning possibilities.

Breaks, cracks, and discontinuous edges display corporal and emotional harm, to humans who've professional maltreatment at the palms of a relative or accomplice.

Tentacles extending outwards from the air of mystery are related with dependency and immaturity, a need for fast gratification and manual. These people are selfish and unreasonable and typically have a tendency to magnify their very very very own importance within the worldwide. They additionally may be energy vampires.

As you develop your talents, you'll see special shapes and deduce their which means that the use of your instinct, expertise, and experience.

We have not however reached the boundaries of our information of auras and the subjects they can display screen. Much of what we recognize about air of secrecy patterns and evaluation is primarily based totally on casual proof and personal revel in, in place of scientific proof, so make sure to hook up with your internal information whilst appearing a reading, and keep an open thoughts.

Ethical Considerations for Aura Interpretation

The exercise of studying the styles of energy that surround the human frame and imparting insights into the bodily, emotional, and religious well-being of human beings is turning into increasingly popular as a device for self-discovery and personal increase. Nevertheless, there are a few important ethical issues to keep in mind even as decoding Auras:

Be excessive quality to have a whole and down to earth understanding of the colors and patterns you could see in an air of secrecy, styles, and what they propose.

Obtain informed consent from the problem of the interpretation. They must understand what it includes, what statistics can be shared, and the way this might impact their lives.

Be humble and aware of the restrictions of charisma interpretation. Do no longer make claims that can not be supported through evidence or revel in.

Be accurate and sincere approximately what your evaluation can also display; presenting fake statistics may additionally need to harm their health and nicely-being.

Maintain confidentiality of the information shared all through an aura interpretation. Respect your subjects' privateness and do no longer proportion records that could be unfavorable to them.

Recommend humans are looking for more steering from medical doctors, counselors, or therapists if there are any troubles approximately their fitness and well-being.

It's important to hold in thoughts those requirements to make sure that charisma interpretation is carried out in a responsible and respectful manner, protective the humans involved. Also, those requirements help to maintain the credibility and legitimacy of this practice, maintaining its charge for personal growth and self-discovery.

Chapter 10: Harmonizing Your Aura

Cleansing Techniques for a Pure Aura

Feeling silly and worn-out is a particular sign you want purification. Keep in thoughts, although, that aura cleansing is right for helping you sense extra efficient, however it is not an alternative to scientific remedy.

The strength from the people round you can affect your strength discipline. Sometimes this has pleasant results, like while you're round someone uplifting and useful. However, there are also some those who are angry, grasping, resentful, or in reality sad, a very good way to have an impact to your air of secrecy, too. If you experience worn-out or sick after spending time with a person, you need to do an air of mystery cleanse.

A gloomy air of thriller is an indication that a few issue is out of alignment; it's a signal of dangerous feelings, on the aspect of greed or anger. Often, you're feeling worn-out or prone, however it can furthermore suggest you're grieving otherwise you're unwell. Cleansing your air of mystery is, over again, critical.

Keeping your air of mystery easy is a outstanding workout due to the truth what you've manifested within the beyond can be nevertheless pending spherical you, and this could now not let you end up the wonderful version of yourself. Without purification, you'll battle to rid your self of feelings of fatigue and oppression.

Cleansing is completed via the usage of the four primary elements:

Water: When you are taking a tub, you're not simply washing your pores and pores and skin – you moreover may additionally clean off the agitation, anger, and energies that aren't yours. Use water to cleanse your power area.

Earth: Even a dust bathtub can easy your pores and pores and pores and skin and your power. This is why they use it in health accommodations or rejuvenation centers.

Air: Gentle wind blowing your clothes and in the course of your face soothes away active muddle and disruption, leaving you feeling apparent and cleansed.

Fire: Can be used as a purifying and recharging approach. Have you ever placed how enjoyable it is to stare right into a campfire? On a smaller scale, you may burn any natural rely and enjoy it inside the equal manner to cleanse your air of mystery and energy.

There are even more precise techniques to smooth or enhance your energy while you're feeling worn-out, overwhelmed, careworn, or unmotivated.

Our thoughts have electricity signatures, which create our worldwide. They supply achievements or failures, possibilities or blockages, melancholy or happiness. Select your thoughts and thoughts with aim. Gather colorful energies round you. This manner you can feel best, and you could select out your choices and movements as it should be.

As you end up greater knowledgeable of the power fields of different people, you'll have a check that someone's deeds, phrases, or mind-set may also carry you up, while others will weaken you. Either lead them, permit them to influence you, or disengage from low-electricity humans.

Choose duties that energize you: crafting, analyzing, taking note of your selected track, dancing, gambling with youngsters and your puppy, or cooking. Be aware at the same time as choosing a career or method that offers you delight.

Enjoy the little miracles of life, your intangible assets. Be smooth, be joyful, and don't fear approximately being criticized. Have some faith in the manner – don't overthink it. Try to stay existence as you want to, even supposing it's in an uncommon way.

At instances on the equal time as you're discouraged, bear in thoughts that there are seasons in existence, and plant life bloom constant with their own agenda. There are only a few guidelines in existence and do now not consciousness on meeting expectations that feel unnatural to you.

A precise diet, proper sleep, adequate exercise, and staying hydrated are critical if you want to characteristic well.

Your environment need to be uplifting. If you're now not feeling top in that you are, try to modify the situation. Learn from those who encourage you, and from individuals who drag you down. Observe nature and spend time outdoors to refresh.

Give yourself time for self-development, for matters that make you sense proud.

Too plenty show time makes you feel slow and fatigued, so disconnect from generation and take breaks from the pc, pill, or phone.

Your electricity state of affairs is a reflected photograph of your inner emotions, so cleaning away awful vibes improves your emotional country. People experience lighter and greater extraordinary and additional real after an aura cleanse. Otherwise, horrible emotions can create obstacles that could distract you from your goals, weighing you down with anger and stress.

Aura cleaning is a personal manner, so follow your intuition.

Transforming Your Aura thru Meditation and Visualization

You are an energetic body, and your air of mystery is proof. It may be seen encircling your frame with colorations indicating which of your chakra energies is advanced.

We want our charisma to be sturdy, to guard us from terrible emotions and energies. A wholesome aura is proof of a sturdy frame, thoughts, and spirit. It allows the development of spiritual abilties and energizes our lives.

Reality is created and modified by means of the thoughts. What you truly don't forget, might be. You can redesign your

Aura via mirrored picture and visualization.

Sit in a meditative posture and ponder for about ten mins to collect your self and interest. Then, within the mind, visualize the power problem around you glowing. Do this for approximately seven extra mins. Visualize a go along with the drift of electricity coming from above and stepping into your Aura from above your head. This power will then nourish and give a boost to your energy field. Do this for another seven mins.

We need to recharge in spirit; this strengthens our energies. Meditation has this impact. We are focusing mindfully to calm the spirit. We connect to higher factors and spirit dimensions, recharging our air of mystery.

Also, mantra meditation is a top notch manner to purify your aura. Choose an incantation that reverberates with you, like "I revel in peace." Sit with out problems and close your eyes, then chant your mantra aloud ten instances. Continue with a five-minute meditation. Direct your mind to your mantra.

You can paintings with your strength issue and chakras via contemplation. Find your self an area in which you could sit down in a comfortable role after which near your eyes. Breathe deeply seven times to lighten up and recognition. Visualize your air of mystery because of the fact the luminous, colorful situation enfolding your frame. Imagine it developing as you breathe deeper. Focus at the crown chakra at the top of your head, or at the coronary coronary heart chakra within the center of your chest. Imagine a whirlwind of power at these locations. As you meditate, watch out for any emotions or emotions that emerge. Give your self sufficient time to begin to experience deeply non violent, and, at the same time as you experience prepared, come once more to reality through using starting your eyes.

Experiment with a few chakra introspection, basing your electricity and connecting your self to the floor. Then, don't forget a cascade of mild discharged throughout you, washing away any strength that you acquired that does not belong to you.

Always keep in thoughts that meditation is a non-public dependancy and there are various proper strategies to do it. Practice and discover what feels most natural and effective to you.

Recharging Your Aura through Energy Work

The diffused existence force electricity is the muse of all existence. It actions via the body and animates us so we will act. It regulates all our abilities. The drift distributes its power thru the frame based on the exceptional and capability of the strength channels and the chakra's energy centers. It moreover impacts our thoughts, emotions, and recognition. Our regular fitness and nicely-being are tied at once to the amount and float of the lifestyles electricity in our frame: it creates strength and energy, it generates the capability for recuperation and well being, it offers us popularity, and it influences our thoughts and as a result affects our potential to meditate.

Our existence electricity comes into the body from our food, the air, and the surroundings. It travels via hundreds of tiny channels to every cellular within the frame, beginning at the bottom of the backbone and going upwards to the pinnacle.

The motion of power is suffering from the location and motion of the body. If you have terrible posture, your breath and energy channels are constricted and the waft of power via your body is diminished. Also, on the equal time as you upward thrust up, power travels upwards toward your head.

The movement of the strength is likewise related with the breath. Inhaling draws the strength upwards and exhaling leads the electricity downward. Breathing strategies manage and domesticate your vital energy and increase your radiance. Also, the quantity and first-rate of strength on your body are crucial to your capability to concentrate. Thoughts will vary with electricity.

So power artwork refers to many practices and techniques aimed towards balancing, shaping, or directing the energy that flows internal and at some point of the frame.

This is the lifestyles force strength, "chi," or "prana" mentioned in a single-of-a-type cultural traditions.

Reiki, acupuncture, qigong, and chakra balancing are some of the strategies to easy imbalances or blockages within the electricity region, which otherwise would possibly in all likelihood result in physical, emotional, or non secular illnesses.

Self-Care for Aura Health and Harmony

You can't do a good deal in existence without the vital electricity. The more dynamic, influencing, and powerful your air of mystery is, the greater active and everyday your achievements in lifestyles can be.

You want to shield your air of thriller. Therefore:

Avoid emotional pollution. Your electricity follows your mind. When your recognition is on high-quality mind and feelings, you feel extra active, happier, and inexperienced. Sometimes it's far essential to break out terrible conduct or take away yourself from a poisonous surroundings. Avoid individuals who are terrible, demanding, or important.

Do breathwork and meditate to free your mind of any poor thoughts and emotional states. Pay interest to the situation of the strength to your body, and shortly it becomes a herbal part of yourself-reputation.

Take brief walks, even in the rain, and study nature to calm your thoughts. Try to get at least a few minutes of light every day; this could enhance your mood and create power – so lie outdoor on a bench, on a blanket, or within the grass, or perform a little gardening to fill your air of mystery with great vibes.

De-muddle. Organize your space and your thoughts – release objects and mind that now not serve you. Don't waste your power on unimportant obligations and permit circulate of things you could't control. Most folks hesitate to allow flow, retaining on even to what didn't education session. But this weakens our energy. Move on from human beings or evaluations that don't upload fee in your life, and get away from negativity and proscribing ideals.

www.ingramcontent.com/pod-product-compliance
Lightning Source LLC
Chambersburg PA
CBHW071439080526
44587CB00014B/1917